Strategies to Protect the Health of DEPLOYED U.S. FORCES

Analytical Framework for Assessing Risks

Lorenz Rhomberg, *Principal Investigator*

Board on Environmental Studies and Toxicology
Commission on Life Sciences
National Research Council

NATIONAL ACADEMY PRESS
Washington, DC

NATIONAL ACADEMY PRESS • 2101 Constitution Ave., N.W. • Washington, D.C. 20418

NOTICE: The project that is the subject of this report was approved by the Governing Board of the National Research Council, whose members are drawn from the councils of the National Academy of Sciences, the National Academy of Engineering, and the Institute of Medicine. The members of the committee responsible for the report were chosen for their special competences and with regard for appropriate balance.

This project was supported by Contract No. DASW01-97-C-0078 between the National Academy of Sciences and the Department of Defense. Any opinions, findings, conclusions, or recommendations expressed in this publication are those of the author(s) and do not necessarily reflect the view of the organizations or agencies that provided support for this project.

International Standard Book Number 0-309-06895-9

Additional copies of this report are available from:

National Academy Press
2101 Constitution Ave., NW
Box 285
Washington, DC 20055
800-624-6242
202-334-3313 (in the Washington metropolitan area)
http://www.nap.edu

Printed in the United States of America

THE NATIONAL ACADEMIES

National Academy of Sciences
National Academy of Engineering
Institute of Medicine
National Research Council

The **National Academy of Sciences** is a private, nonprofit, self-perpetuating society of distinguished scholars engaged in scientific and engineering research, dedicated to the furtherance of science and technology and to their use for the general welfare. Upon the authority of the charter granted to it by the Congress in 1863, the Academy has a mandate that requires it to advise the federal government on scientific and technical matters. Dr. Bruce M. Alberts is president of the National Academy of Sciences.

The **National Academy of Engineering** was established in 1964, under the charter of the National Academy of Sciences, as a parallel organization of outstanding engineers. It is autonomous in its administration and in the selection of its members, sharing with the National Academy of Sciences the responsibility for advising the federal government. The National Academy of Engineering also sponsors engineering programs aimed at meeting national needs, encourages education and research, and recognizes the superior achievements of engineers. Dr. William A. Wulf is president of the National Academy of Engineering.

The **Institute of Medicine** was established in 1970 by the National Academy of Sciences to secure the services of eminent members of appropriate professions in the examination of policy matters pertaining to the health of the public. The Institute acts under the responsibility given to the National Academy of Sciences by its congressional charter to be an adviser to the federal government and, upon its own initiative, to identify issues of medical care, research, and education. Dr. Kenneth I. Shine is president of the Institute of Medicine.

The **National Research Council** was organized by the National Academy of Sciences in 1916 to associate the broad community of science and technology with the Academy's purposes of furthering knowledge and advising the federal government. Functioning in accordance with general policies determined by the Academy, the Council has become the principal operating agency of both the National Academy of Sciences and the National Academy of Engineering in providing services to the government, the public, and the scientific and engineering communities. The Council is administered jointly by both Academies and the Institute of Medicine. Dr. Bruce M. Alberts and Dr. William A. Wulf are chairman and vice chairman, respectively, of the National Research Council.

PRINCIPAL INVESTIGATOR

Lorenz Rhomberg, Gradient Corporation, Cambridge, Massachusetts (formerly of Harvard School of Public Health, Boston, Massachusetts)

ADVISORY GROUP

Arthur J. Barsky, Brigham and Women's Hospital, Boston, Massachusetts
Germaine M. Buck, State University of New York at Buffalo, Buffalo, New York
William S. Cain, University of California, San Diego, California
John Doull, The University of Kansas Medical Center, Kansas City, Kansas
Ernest Hodgson, North Carolina State University, Raleigh, North Carolina
David H. Moore, Battelle Memorial Institute, Bel Air, Maryland
Roy Reuter, Life Systems, Inc., Cleveland, Ohio
Ken W. Sexton, University of Minnesota, Minneapolis, Minnesota
Robert E. Shope, University of Texas, Medical Branch, Galveston, Texas
Ainsley Weston, National Institute of Occupational Safety and Health, Morgantown, West Virginia

Staff

Carol A. Maczka, Project Director
Raymond A. Wassel, Program Director
Susan N.J. Pang, Program Officer
Robert J. Crossgrove, Editor
Norman Grossblatt, Editor
Catherine M. Kubik, Senior Project Assistant
Leah L. Probst, Project Assistant
Mirsada Karalic-Loncarevic, Information Specialist

Sponsor

U.S. Department of Defense

COMMISSION ON LIFE SCIENCES

OTHER REPORTS OF THE BOARD ON ENVIRONMENTAL STUDIES AND TOXICOLOGY

Waste Incineration and Public Health (1999)
Hormonally Active Agents in the Environment (1999)
Research Priorities for Airborne Particulate Matter: II. Evaluating Research Progress and Updating the Portfolio (1999)
Ozone-Forming Potential of Reformulated Gasoline (1999)
Risk-Based Waste Classification in California (1999)
Arsenic in Drinking Water (1999)
Research Priorities for Airborne Particulate Matter: I. Immediate Priorities and a Long-Range Research Portfolio (1998)
Brucellosis in the Greater Yellowstone Area (1998)
The National Research Council's Committee on Toxicology: The First 50 Years (1997)
Toxicologic Assessment of the Army's Zinc Cadmium Sulfide Dispersion Tests (1997)
Carcinogens and Anticarcinogens in the Human Diet (1996)
Upstream: Salmon and Society in the Pacific Northwest (1996)
Science and the Endangered Species Act (1995)
Wetlands: Characteristics and Boundaries (1995)
Biologic Markers (5 reports, 1989-1995)
Review of EPA's Environmental Monitoring and Assessment Program (3 reports, 1994-1995)
Science and Judgment in Risk Assessment (1994)
Ranking Hazardous Waste Sites for Remedial Action (1994)
Pesticides in the Diets of Infants and Children (1993)
Issues in Risk Assessment (1993)
Setting Priorities for Land Conservation (1993)
Protecting Visibility in National Parks and Wilderness Areas (1993)
Dolphins and the Tuna Industry (1992)
Hazardous Materials on the Public Lands (1992)
Science and the National Parks (1992)
Animals as Sentinels of Environmental Health Hazards (1991)
Assessment of the U.S. Outer Continental Shelf Environmental Studies Program, Volumes I-IV (1991-1993)
Human Exposure Assessment for Airborne Pollutants (1991)
Monitoring Human Tissues for Toxic Substances (1991)
Rethinking the Ozone Problem in Urban and Regional Air Pollution (1991)
Decline of the Sea Turtles (1990)

Copies of these reports may be ordered from the National Academy Press
(800) 624-6242
(202) 334-3313
www.nap.edu

Preface

Illnesses possibly associated with U.S. military deployments during Operations Desert Storm and Desert Shield (1990-1991) have been the subject of much debate and national attention. In order to help prevent and reduce the number of illnesses in future deployments, the Department of Defense (DOD) requested that the National Academy of Sciences (NAS) develop a long-term strategy for protecting the health of the nation's military personnel when deployed to unfamiliar environments. As part of the academy's response to this request, I was asked to develop an analytical framework for assessing risks to deployed forces from a variety of health threats encountered during deployments. A group of advisers was convened to assist me with the project, providing me with advice in their various areas of expertise and guiding the development of the framework. I am very appreciative of the valuable input they provided.

As part of the information gathering for this study, DOD personnel provided very useful presentations on relevant DOD programs. I wish to acknowledge in particular COL Francis O'Donnell (Office of the Special Assistant for Gulf War Illness), Jack Heller (U.S. Army Center for Health Promotion and Preventive Medicine), John Resta (U.S. Army Center for Health Promotion and Preventive Medicine), Hank Gardner (U.S. Army Center for Environmental Health Research), MAJ Larry Kimm (Joint Staff), CDR Paul Knechtges (U.S. Army Center for Environmental Health Research), and Thomas Burke (Johns Hopkins University). These briefings were especially helpful because I was chosen for this project expressly as a person without extensive experience in military matters and am not well versed in military organization structure, operations, policy, or doctrine. Since DOD's aim was specifically to obtain an independent assessment of how the military can protect their deployed personnel in the future, I hope my newness to these matters can lead to some benefit in freshness of point of view that will offset the lack of extensive experience into the military's current extensive activities and programs.

Special thanks are owed to the six authors who were commissioned to write papers on topics that needed more in-depth analysis. Morton Lippmann (New York University School of Medicine) discussed approaches for collecting and using personal exposure and biological-marker information for assessing health risks; Edward Martin (Edward Martin and Associates, Inc.) characterized possible scenarios of future deployments and battle considerations; Joseph Rodricks (The Life Sciences Consultancy) reviewed traditional risk assessment methods and how risk assessment in general might be applied to deployment scenarios; Joan Rose (University of South Florida) addressed health assessment and risk management integration for biological agents; Karl Rozman (University of Kansas Medical Center) proposed a new paradigm for incorporating toxicokinetic information in risk assessment; and Raymond Yang (Colorado State University) discussed toxicologic interactions among harmful agents. These authoritative papers were presented at a workshop on January 28-29, 1999 in Washington, DC, and have been published concurrently with this report (see *Workshop Proceedings on Strategies to Protect the Health of Deployed U.S. Forces: Assessing Health Risks to Deployed U.S. Forces*).

This report has been reviewed in draft form by individuals chosen for their technical expertise and diverse perspectives in accordance with procedures approved by the NRC's Report Review Committee for reviewing NRC and Institute of Medicine reports. The purpose of that independent review was to provide candid and critical comments to assist the NRC in making the published report as sound as possible and to ensure that the report meets institutional standards for objectivity, evidence, and responsiveness to the study charge. The review comments and draft manuscript remain confidential to protect the integrity of the deliberative process. I wish to thank the following individuals, who are neither officials nor employees of the NRC, for their participation in the review of this report: John C. Bailar, III, University of Chicago; Thomas A. Burke, Johns Hopkins University; Steven D. Colome, Irvine, California; John L. Emmerson, Fishers, Indiana; Bernard D. Goldstein, Rutgers University; Rogene F. Henderson, Lovelace Respiratory Research Institute; Peter Hidalgo, Waverly Hall, Georgia; Paul Knechtges, Sherikon, Inc.; Matthew S. Meselson, Harvard University; and Arthur C. Upton, Rutgers University.

The individuals listed above, as well as the advisers for this project, have provided many constructive comments and suggestions. It must be emphasized, however, that responsibility for the final content of this report rests entirely with the principal investigator and the NRC.

I would also like to acknowledge the principal investigators of the three sister projects that were conducted concurrently with this one. Thomas McKone (University of California, Berkeley) was the principal investigator of a project that considered technology and methods for detection and tracking of exposures to a subset of harmful agents; Michael Kleinman (University of California, Irvine) and Michael Wartell (Indiana University - Purdue University Fort Wayne) were co-investigators of a project that reviewed and evaluated approaches and technologies used in the development and evaluation of equipment and clothing for physical protection and decontamination; and Samuel Guze (Washington University) and Phillip Russell were co-investigators who reviewed and evaluated medical protection, health consequences management and treatment, and medical record keeping.

My personal thanks are also owed to the NRC staff who were involved in this project. In particular, Carol A. Maczka and Raymond A. Wassel expertly brought structure to the project and guided the interactions among DOD briefers, the advisory committee, and the commissioned authors along productive lines. Susan N.J. Pang provided essential technical help, especially in obtaining documentation and preparing material. Other staff members who contributed to this effort are James J. Reisa, Robert J. Crossgrove, Catherine M. Kubik, and Leah L. Probst.

Lorenz Rhomberg
Principal Investigator

Contents

Strategies to Protect the Health of DEPLOYED U.S. FORCES

Analytical Framework for Assessing Risks

Executive Summary

Deployment of forces in hostile or unfamiliar environments is inherently risky. The changing missions and increasing use of U.S. forces around the globe in operations other than battle call for greater attention to threats of non-battle-related health problems—including infections, pathogen- and vector-borne diseases, exposure to toxicants, and psychological and physical stress—all of which must be avoided or treated differently from battle casualties. The likelihood of exposure to chemical and biological weapons adds to the array of tactical threats against which protection is required. The health consequences of physical and psychological stress, by themselves or through interaction with other threats, are also increasingly recognized. In addition, the military's responsibility in examining potential health and safety risks to its troops is increasing, and the spectrum of health concerns is broadening, from acute illness and injury due to pathogens and accidents to possible influences of low-level chemical exposures, which can manifest themselves in reproductive health and chronic illnesses years later, perhaps even after cessation of military service.

Some well-publicized cases have led to scrutiny of the military's procedures for identifying potential hazards and for collecting the information on hazards, exposure, and health-status surveillance that is necessary to detect and monitor threats to the troops' health and welfare.

To help prevent and reduce the number of illnesses in future deployments, the Department of Defense (DOD) asked the National Academy of Sciences (NAS) to advise it on a long-term strategy for protecting the health of the nation's military personnel when deployed to unfamiliar environments. In response to this request, a collaborative effort was established between the Institute of Medicine (IOM) and the National Research Council (NRC) and four tasks were identified as key to addressing DOD's request. They were: (1) develop an analytical framework for assessing health risks to deployed forces; (2) review and evaluate technology and methods for detection and tracking of exposures to potentially harmful chemical and biological agents; (3) review and evaluate technology and methods for physical protection and decontamination, particularly of chemical and biological agents; and (4) review and evaluate medical protection, health consequences management and treatment, and medical record keeping.

This report addresses the first task of developing an analytical framework for assessing risks, which would encompass the risks of adverse health effects from battle injuries, including those from chemical- and biological-warfare agents, and the non-battle-related health problems noted above. The presumed spectrum of deployment ranged from peacekeeping to full-scale conflict.

APPROACH TO THE CHARGE

This report was prepared by Dr. Lorenz Rhomberg of Gradient Corporation (formerly of the Harvard School of Public Health), with the help and guidance of 10 advisers who represented various scientific disciplines, including military operations, toxicology, infectious diseases, use of biomarkers, personal exposure assessment, epidemiology, occupational health, psychiatry, and risk assessment (see Appendix B). The group received briefings, reviewed documentation of current DOD practices, considered existing risk-assessment paradigms, and commissioned the preparation of papers on six topics that required in-depth analyses (see Appendix A for abstracts of these papers).

The focus of this report is principally on risk assessment—the identification, characterization, and quantitative description of threats and the impacts they may produce—rather than on the means to control or manage those impacts. It must be borne in mind, however, that such risk assessment must occur within the military context, aimed at enhancing the health and safety of troops while ensuring their military effectiveness, both strategically (through improvement of equipment, doctrine, training, and preparedness) and in actions taken during specific deployments. While the risk assessment framework recommended in this report does not directly address how to put its characterizations of threats to use in risk management decision-making, it does attempt to steer the conduct of risk assessment activities so as to provide the most useful and appropriate information while avoiding critical gaps.

Because of the diversity of threats that the recommended framework must be able to address, it cannot be very specific about any one activity, and it does not try to be a flowchart or decision tree that maps out a process, step by step. The term "framework" as used herein means an organized context for conducting assessment activities that defines the relationship of the component activities to the achievement of the larger aims of protecting the health of deployed forces. Rather than a prescription of a specific program or a plan for its implementation, the framework is a set of strategies for conducting risk assessment activities so as to be most useful to the military's needs. Accordingly, emphasis is placed on examining how those needs differ from the more widely familiar context of environmental risk assessment. The NRC's 1983 risk-assessment paradigm forms the core of the framework, providing a structure for analysis and characterization of particular exposures to particular hazards. The framework recommended herein expands the scope of the paradigm, by showing that the structure can address not only toxic chemicals, but also such other threats as risks of microbial infections, mechanical failures, transportation accidents, and tactical threats. The particular technical methods will vary with the nature of the threat under analysis, and the framework includes ways of modifying standard approaches to be applicable to military situations.

The framework must go beyond the NRC paradigm to organize the process of recognizing how the varied activities entailed in deployment of forces might lead to exposures to hazards that need analysis, cataloging these, setting priorities among them for analysis, analyzing them, and integrating the results so as to yield a comprehensive risk-management program that addresses the full array of threats with which troops must deal during deployment.

Threats to deployed forces can be assessed with the tools developed in the civilian risk-assessment context, but it must be recognized that the military context differs. Many hazards are specific to military situations, military exposure factors can differ from those relevant to civilians, and stress and extreme environments can affect toxic responses. A useful management scheme must address all the threats that deployed troops face, so integration is particularly needed. The military mission has primacy, and its needs might dictate that troops bear risks that would not be acceptable in a civilian setting. Extraordinary measures to protect against threats to health and safety can encumber military effectiveness or increase vulnerability, so well-thought-out tradeoffs among military and nonmilitary concerns are necessary. Risk information must be presented in a way that permits rapid decisions to be made in the field by commanders with little pertinent technical expertise.

For many hazards relevant to military deployments, the concern is not for continuous low-level exposures, but for episodes that occur as a consequence of unplanned and unpredictable events, such as equipment failures, actions by an adversary, and collateral damage of chemical-storage facilities. Risk analysis for such hazards must focus as much on describing the likelihood of toxicologically important exposures as on the responses to exposures. One can analyze such exposures by tracing scenarios leading to exposure of troops and by examining the likelihood that key precipitating events occur, whether they be physical occurrences or actions on the part of adversaries or of the deployed forces themselves. The problem can often be divided into the likelihood that a potential hazard is in the deployment area, the likelihood of release of a hazard into the environment, the likelihood of exposure of troops to the released material (based on fate and transport modeling), and the likelihood of adverse health effects, given the exposure (based on dose-response analysis).

No attempt is made in this report to assess particular individual risks or to critique the current DOD systems or established risk-assessment practices, nor is any attempt made to create a comprehensive catalog of threats. The risks of injury from conventional weapons or nuclear weapons are not addressed herein, and psychological stress is addressed only in general, because of the lack of established ways to assess the risk of such stress. This omission is a shortcoming of the risk assessment framework recommended in this report, since psychological stress is a factor of major importance to the health of deployed forces and deployment veterans, and any solution to how DOD should approach disorders and unexplained symptoms among veterans must include consideration of the contribution of stress. Further work on this topic is recommended.

A risk-assessment framework should be a means to help achieve DOD's program objectives for addressing the health and safety risks to deployed forces, so such objectives must be clearly defined. It is provisionally suggested that they should include minimizing the impact of disease and non-battle-related injuries; developing a straightforward and systematic program to address risks and executing the program efficiently; diligently and competently addressing health and safety threats; integrating risk awareness and the appropriate weighing of risks and benefits into decision-making; improving the ability to characterize risks posed by past exposures; and doing all the foregoing in the light of cost and effects on military capability and effectiveness. The recommended framework attempts to bring the methodology of risk assessment to bear on these objectives.

The process should be open, encouraging scrutiny of DOD actions and the incorporation of health and safety concerns into all aspects of decision-making. Emphasis should be placed on proactive recognition of potential threats, and charxèterizing and setting priorities for them; monitoring for detection and characterization of known threats and their impacts; and ongoing and retrospective surveillance of troops' (and veterans') health status for effects that may arise despite protective efforts.

DESCRIPTION OF THE FRAMEWORK

The recommended framework is a structured approach to gathering, organizing, and analyzing information in a way that encourages a comprehensive, integrative assessment and response to the threats that deployed troops might face. Unlike more traditional risk assessments, the recommended framework is concerned with examining *activities* (such as deployment near an industrial facility that stores various toxic chemicals) rather than *specific threats*. Focusing on the threats associated with particular military deployment activities, rather than specific threats, encourages thinking beyond a standard list of recognized hazards, facilitates redesign of practices and materiel to mitigate risks, and avoids increasing one risk to reduce another. By emphasizing planning and attention to previously uncharacterized threats, the framework aims to minimize the likelihood of overlooking important risk factors. Characterizing the effects of various levels of exposure, as opposed to simply defining "safe" levels, increases the ability to make appropriate tradeoffs.

The recommended framework for risk assessment of threats to deployed U.S. forces is composed of three phases, which are characterized by the timeline of deployment: ongoing, deployment, and post-deployment (see Table E-1).

TABLE E-1 Framework for Phases of Risk Assessment

Ongoing Strategic Baseline Preparation
Anticipation of potential threats and circumstances
Priority-setting for detailed analyses
Risk analysis
Incorporation of results into planning
During Deployment
Deployment-specific planning
Initial activities
Continued deployment
Activities to terminate deployment
Post-deployment
Reintegration of troops
Data archiving
Continuing health surveillance
Population analyses of exposure effects
Evaluation of lessons learned

Ongoing Strategic Preparation

The ongoing strategic baseline preparation phase of the framework involves all the activities and analyses undertaken to prepare for threats in future deployments. The activities are not tied to particular deployments, but represent the need for continuing development of information about potential deployment risks and exposures, organized through the framework so as to create an ever expanding and improving base of knowledge. This knowledge can be drawn upon to increase the capability to avoid or mitigate risk and to refine doctrine and training so as to lead to safer deployments.

Ongoing preparation has four steps: anticipating potential threats and the circumstances under which they might arise, setting priorities among the potential threats for analysis, conducting qualitative and quantitative risk analyses of the threats, and incorporating the resulting risk estimates into exposure guidelines and planning. In the first step, established lists of hazardous threats (such as toxic chemicals, infectious disease agents, insecticides, and vaccines) are reviewed, and threats with notable exposure patterns are examined. Potential threats can be identified by constructing deployment scenarios and placing hazards in three categories: those associated with deployment-specific activities (such as heat stress), those associated with particular types of missions (such as peace-keeping and ground combat), and those associated with particular locations (such as climate, indigenous diseases, and local pollution). In addition to identifying potential exposures to threats, the scenario-drawing process helps to link exposures directly to the activities that cause them and to delineate chains of events that lead to particular outcomes. It is important to consider in this step the potential for coexposures (such as vaccinations, antidotes, and pesticides) that could lead to accumulative or synergistic effects.

Once the potential threats to deployed troops are identified, priorities must be set for analysis. That is done by examining the most likely deployment scenarios and determining which hazards are most likely, which are mission-critical (would affect the chance of success of the military mission), which constitute known threats, which could have widespread or severe effects, and which are peculiar to the deployment setting—all features that suggest priority attention.

Once the hazards and the circumstances under which they might arise are identified and ranked, the traditional tools of risk assessment can be used to develop quantitative or qualitative risk estimates. In the dose-response analysis, consideration should be given to potential interactions with other threats, the duration of exposure, and the importance of dose-rate effects. For each potential hazard, it is also important to examine the possible scenarios that lead to an adverse outcome and to recognize that some scenarios require a chain of events to produce the outcome, in which case the probability of each scenario is based on the probabilities of the separate events.

An important step in the ongoing strategic baseline preparation phase of the framework is the incorporation of the risk-assessment results into planning, design of doctrine and standard operating procedures, and training. For example, exposure standards can be established for achieving some degree of protection under different circumstances (such as short-term emergency exposures and chronic low-level exposures). Because detailed risk analysis can be time-consuming, appropriate generic analyses and contingency plans that can quickly be adapted to and implemented in actual deployment situations should be formulated. Such formulations should take account of the fact that different deployment missions will have different spectra of tactical risk, as well as different opportunities and costs for health protective measures.

During Deployment

The second major phase of the framework addresses risk-assessment activities associated with actual specific deployments, either as case-specific pre-deployment planning preparation or as activities conducted during the course of deployment. The key activities associated with this phase are implementing plans made in anticipation of deployment (ongoing strategic baseline preparation and planning), refining them with information peculiar to the specific deployment, noting the advent of threatening exposures, and activating the appropriate parts of the response plans accordingly. This phase must also include vigilance for exposures that, despite all the planning, were unanticipated. DOD should examine the effectiveness of collecting and archiving biological samples, in addition to sera, from troops and environmental samples for future analysis. Such information could provide rapid results during deployment so that risk management can be continually refined. This information could also validate and refine baseline strategies.

When a specific deployment is expected, information on its location, mission, and current conditions should be incorporated into predesigned generalized contingency plans. This includes information on meteorological conditions and forecasts, updates on the locations of hazardous materials, and current assessments of capabilities and inclinations of adversaries. A plan to obtain information on potential exposures during the course of deployment should be specified; its extent will depend on the nature, magnitude, and anticipated duration of the specific deployment. On arrival at a deployment destination, samples of soil, air, and water should be obtained and tested for local pollutants, and some samples should be archived for future reference. In addition, detection devices for the most likely threats and meteorological instruments should be set up to obtain information for use in exposure models.

Over the course of the deployment, various kinds of information should be collected periodically (with the extent of the activity depending on the deployment specifics): environmental samples to document changes in environmental concentrations, information on unit activities and positions, and information collected by monitors and detectors. DOD should examine the effectiveness and feasibility of collecting biological samples during deployment. It is also important during the course of deployment to be vigilant for novel and unanticipated threats.

The information collected during deployment is valuable for retrospective analyses, such as reconstruction of exposure scenarios, comparisons with pre-deployment health surveys and samples, and improvement in contingency plans. These data constitute an important source of information for investigating health issues that might arise among deployment veterans.

After Deployment

Post-deployment risk assessment is the third major phase of the framework. In this phase, the health of deployment veterans is monitored for later-appearing effects, and analyses are conducted to ascertain whether these effects are associated with exposures experienced during deployment.

DOD should consider the effectiveness of collecting and archiving health information and biological samples after deployment for the purpose of follow-up and retrospective analyses to address questions about illnesses that might arise later. Surveillance of veterans' health should be continued, and uncertain outcomes should be investigated with exposure reconstruction and epidemiologic analyses. Much of the information obtained about threats during this phase of the framework can be used to refine the ongoing strategic baseline risk analyses by providing a deeper understanding of known threats and by identifying threats not previously considered.

RECOMMENDATIONS

The risk-assessment framework presented in this report should be used by DOD as a basis for organizing its efforts and learning what kinds of work are needed for the protection of the safety and health of forces deployed in hostile environments.

What will make the framework most useful is not the execution of each of its elements, however competently done, but rather the systematic approach to the process of assessing threats to deployed troops and incorporating the results of each element of analysis into an integrated program that addresses the overall objectives of the troop health-protection program.

In implementing the framework, DOD should

- Develop an explicit list of objectives, such as those described in this report, for efforts to protect the health and safety of deployed forces and to periodically assess progress in meeting the objectives.
- Strive to examine and reexamine as warranted all the effects of a given hazardous agent or threat, not only the effects that were first known, including risks posed by low exposures that could eventually lead to chronic illness.
- Continue to conduct research on methods to address different magnitudes, durations, patterns, and coexposures that might be encountered during deployment.
- Develop risk-assessment methods to characterize and predict effects of psychological and physical stress in potentiating or exacerbating the physical, chemical, and biological effects of hazardous agents or threats and as hazards in their own right.
- Conduct research and develop methods to assess risks posed by exposure to microbial agents, and strive to characterize the variety of disease organisms that might be encountered around the world and troops' vulnerability to them.
- Examine patterns of coexposure to various threats; because deployment is characterized by many simultaneous exposures, develop methods to assess possible effects of combinations of threats and their interactions with stress; and develop methods to identify the combinations that should receive further scrutiny based upon biological considerations, because they are peculiar to specific kinds of deployment, or because of particular DOD responsibilities.
- Make special efforts to identify previously unrecognized hazards by examining deployment activities and settings for potential threats and by identifying scenarios that might lead to hazardous exposures.
- As an aid to decision-making in emergencies related to particular hazardous substances, compile and make readily accessible the exposure levels and durations at which people are expected to begin to suffer progressively severe effects.
- Conduct expert analyses before deployment to update general scenarios with case-specific details for quick application by field commanders.

- Conduct research on developing appropriate biological markers of exposure and effect for surveillance of exposures that are of particular relevance to the deployment setting.
- As part of the tracking of troops' exposures and activities, DOD should consider the effectiveness of collecting and archiving biological samples, in addition to sera, from troops and environmental samples before, during (if warranted and feasible), and after deployment.
- Conduct annual health evaluations of reserve and active-duty personnel to obtain baseline health information, as recommended in the companion IOM report addressing medical surveillance.
- Develop an explicit framework for risk-management decision-making that would use information obtained from the application of the risk-assessment framework.

1

Introduction

Recent wars and conflicts, such as Operations Desert Shield and Desert Storm, have highlighted the need for the U.S. military to protect its forces from a variety of health threats associated with deployment, including those indirectly related to battle. In this report, the term "deployment" is defined as "A troop movement resulting from a [Joint Chiefs of Staff]/unified command deployment order for 30 continuous days or greater to a land-based location outside the United States that does not have a permanent U.S. military medical treatment facility" (JCS 1998). Following the Persian Gulf War, in which there were few casualties, a large number of unanticipated and still undiagnosed illnesses developed that caused many veterans of that conflict to express concerns about possible exposures to hazardous materials and other potential risk factors associated with their deployment. As a result, a number of task forces and committees, such as the Defense Science Board Task Force on Persian Gulf War Effects, the Office of the Special Assistant for Gulf War Illnesses, and the Presidential Advisory Committee on Gulf War Veterans' Illnesses, were established and devoted to examining those concerns. The principal focus of those efforts has been on understanding the current health of veterans, ensuring appropriate evaluation and care of veterans' health concerns, and determining connections between service in the Persian Gulf and specific exposures and the veterans' current health status.

To help prevent and reduce the number of unanticipated illnesses in future deployments, the Department of Defense (DOD) requested that the National Academy of Sciences (NAS) advise DOD on a long-term strategy for protecting the health of the nation's military personnel when deployed to unfamiliar environments. In response to this request, a collaborative effort was established between the Institute of Medicine (IOM) and the National Research Council (NRC) and four tasks were identified as key to addressing DOD's request. These are as follows: (1) develop an analytical framework for assessing health risks to deployed forces; (2) review and evaluate technology and methods for detection and tracking of exposures to potentially harmful chemical and biological agents; (3) review and evaluate technology and methods for physical protection and decontamination, particularly of chemical and biological agents; and (4) review and evaluate medical protection, health consequences management and treatment, and medical record keeping.

The tasks were carried out by principal investigators with the help and guidance of panels of expert advisers and with an understanding of DOD's need to make trade-offs or set acceptable levels of risk. The risk of injury from conventional weapons or nuclear weapons was not considered. The presumed spectrum of conflict in which exposures could occur in the future ranged from peacekeeping to full-scale conflict. The principal investigators collaborated and had the opportunity to attend the meetings and briefings of the other tasks. Separate reports on each task were published concurrently (see NRC 1999a,b and IOM 1999). This report addresses the first task, which is described more fully below.

ASSESSING HEALTH RISKS TO DEPLOYED FORCES

Assessment of the risk of disease and other health outcomes in military personnel requires specific information on potential causative factors, exposure scenarios, dose-response relationships, and types of health responses expected from contact with an agent, mixtures, or sequences of potentially harmful agents. The purpose of this task was to develop an analytical framework that would facilitate the assessment of such risks to deployed forces. The risks that were considered were those incurred from battle injuries, especially from chemical-warfare and biological-warfare agents, and from disease and non-battle injuries (DNBI). DNBI-producing agents include infectious diseases, psychological stress, heat and cold injuries, and unintentional injuries. In developing the analytical framework, information and approaches to addressing the following issues were considered: (1) characterization of sources and releases of specific potentially harmful agents and their transport and fate in all environmental media (air, water, and soil); (2) identification of important routes of exposure (inhalation, dermal absorption, ingestion of liquids, and consumption of food), and concentrations of agents at the point of exposure; (3) determination of exposure scenarios and resulting exposures among populations of military personnel; and (4) identification of the types of acute and chronic health responses (e.g., neurological effects, immunological effects, reproductive effects, cancer, and infectious disease) under a variety of environmental and physiological conditions (including extreme temperatures and psychological stress) that could be predicted based on toxicological and epidemiological information, exposure-health response relationships, and possible interactions among harmful agents themselves and with administered drugs. Health responses among various sensitive or susceptible subpopulations were also considered.

In addition to developing a health risk-assessment framework, approaches for implementing the framework were considered. Approaches included appropriate use of tools, such as biological markers and other techniques, methods for relating toxicological, toxicokinetic, and toxicodynamic information observed from animal testing and other studies to the prediction of causal relationships in humans, estimation of human exposure levels, use of assumptions when data gaps exist, measures to assess uncertainty, and use of various quantitative methods, such as probabilistic models.

THE APPROACH TO THE TASK

Focusing the Task

The request to NAS was to develop an analytical framework for assessing risks from a broad array of threats, including battle injuries, chemical and biological warfare agents, diseases, and non-battle injuries connected with deployment. Included in these threats are the risks of acute and chronic health effects from exposures to chemicals associated with deployment tasks (including prophylactic treatments and protective agents and measures, such as pesticides, that are brought to the theatre by the deployment force itself), as well as those that might be encountered in the deployment environment. How these threats might interact and how physical and psychological stress might affect them are also highly relevant, as is the question of such stresses themselves being threats.

Depending on how this task is defined, the magnitude of the undertaking is potentially enormous. Troops might be sent to many different areas of the world on many different missions, and each deployment will face a different and complex array of threats. The catalog of potential threats is vast, their nature is highly diverse, and the technical approaches needed to address them span a wide array of scientific disciplines. The potential circumstances of exposure are virtually infinite, varying with the setting, the nature of the deployment, and the activities of the troops. It is also critical to acknowledge that, in the military setting, some risks must be borne in furtherance of essential military missions, and so the question of balancing health and safety risks with the needs of the mission must be part of the approach.

Finally, one could read DOD's charge as calling for a comprehensive review, critique, redesign, and plan for the implementation of the whole body of efforts at DOD touching on the health and safety of troops in and out of combat. In view of this, the first need in the development of a framework for assessing risks is to refine and focus the scope of the task.

Two broad themes—one practical and one conceptual—tie together the analysis of the wide variety of threats to deployed forces. The practical one is that a program to protect the health of deployed troops must strive to consider all sources of potential impact. The assessments of individual sources of risk must in the end come together into a comprehensive risk-management program that includes how to behave in the face of the whole array of threats, avoid or ameliorate those threats, balance some risks against others, and weigh achieving mission objectives without entailing unnecessary risks. Thus, despite the diversity of threats and the different technical approaches that might be appropriate to characterize them, they cannot effectively be managed in isolation from one another. A common framework is needed to provide a basis for comparisons among threats and the integration of results into a well-reasoned program of risk management.

The conceptual theme that ties analysis of diverse threats together is the paradigm of risk analysis. Despite the diversity in the causes and nature of the threats, each threat represents a set of potential degrees of loss that might or might not happen, with the uncertainty in outcome arising not only from incomplete knowledge of the underlying causes but also from the unknown course of future events. Analysis can help characterize the array of the possible degrees of loss and the likelihood of occurrence of each loss. This conceptual paradigm provides a means to achieve the practical need for integration of results referred to above. A deployment risk-assessment framework should also provide a basis for investigating and comparing the potential costs and benefits of alternative decisions and under different scenarios in a way that acknowledges the uncertainties. In this analysis, it is possible to consider the array of potential hazards, the degree of certainty with which those hazards are known and characterized, the potential for additional information to clarify uncertainties, the likelihood that troops will be challenged by the threat in practice, and the possible extent of impact on their health that might result.

Clearly, a framework for assessing risks must also address the goals of the overall enterprise. Risk analysis must include organization, summarization, and presentation of information, done with the motivating questions in mind. Chapter 2 proposes objectives for a risk-assessment framework that emphasize the need not only to characterize recognized risks, but also to carry out a systematic examination of deployment activities to bring to light heretofore unrecognized threats. This examination should also maintain due diligence toward the responsibility of the military for the health and safety of deployed troops.

The focus of this report is principally on risk assessment—the identification, characterization, and quantitative description of threats and the impacts they may produce—rather than on the means to control or manage those impacts. It must be borne in mind, however, that this assessment occurs within the larger context of the DOD's activities aimed at enhancing the health and safety of troops while ensuring their military effectiveness, both strategically (through improvement of equipment, doctrine, training, and preparedness) and in actions taken during specific deployments. While the framework does not directly address how to put its characterizations of threats to use in these decision-making contexts, it does attempt to steer the conduct of risk assessment activities so as to provide the most useful and appropriate information while avoiding critical gaps.

Because of the diversity of analyses the framework must cover, it cannot be very specific about any one activity, and it does not try to be a flowchart or decision tree that maps out a process step by step. By "framework," the present report means an organized context for conducting assessment activities that defines the relationship of the component activities to the achievement of the larger aims of protecting the health of deployed forces. Rather than a prescription of a specific program or a plan for its implementation, the framework is a set of strategies for conducting risk assessment activities so as to be most useful to the military's needs. Accordingly, stress is put on examining how those needs differ from the more widely familiar context of environmental risk assessment.

In sum, the approach to defining a framework for risk assessment over the broad array of threats should be one that emphasizes a systematic approach to cataloguing and assessing the various kinds and sources of hazard, encourages attention to the question of unrecognized threats, and approaches the analysis of each kind of threat in the commonality paradigm of risk analysis.

Methods

In developing the framework, a number of factors and trends were examined that bear on the changing context for risk analysis, and the particular challenges faced by the military, which together prompt a closer examination of what the military can and should do to protect the health and safety of deployed forces. In addition, existing frameworks were examined for their usefulness according to a set of stated objectives and the special needs and aspects of U.S. troop deployment.

The development of this framework did not rely solely on following the more traditional structure of focusing on a list of recognized toxic agents, assessing their potencies, describing likely exposure scenarios, characterizing the consequences of these exposures, and investigating what changes in practice might avoid or mitigate the risks. Instead, the approach focused on a framework that examines how the various activities, actions, and settings of deployment come to present threats, how likely it is that threats will be manifested, and how mitigating one risk might raise others.

The task of developing an analytical framework for assessing risks was carried out by a principal investigator with the help and guidance of a panel of 10 advisers, who represented such diverse disciplines as military operations, toxicology, infectious diseases, biomarkers, personal exposure assessment, epidemiology, occupational health, psychiatry, and risk assessment. This panel considered a vast amount of information, including briefings and documentation of current risk assessments provided by DOD, existing risk-assessment paradigms, and six detailed papers commissioned specifically for this task on topics that the principal investigator and advisers identified as needing in-depth analyses. These commissioned papers were presented at a workshop on January 28-29, 1999, in Washington, D.C.: "Approaches for the Collection and Use of Personal Exposure and Human Biological-Marker Information for Assessing Risks to Deployed U.S. Forces," by Morton Lippmann; "Characteristics of the Future Battlefield and Deployment," by Edward Martin; "The Nature of Risk Assessment and its Application to Deployed U.S. Forces," by Joseph Rodricks; "Future Health Assessment and Risk Management Integration for Infectious Diseases and Biological Weapons for Deployed U.S. Forces," by Joan Rose; "Approaches for Using Toxicokinetic Information in Assessing Risks to Deployed U.S. Forces," by Karl Rozman; and "Health Risks and Preventive Research Strategy for Deployed U.S. Forces from Toxicologic Interactions Among Potentially Harmful Agents," by Raymond Yang. See Appendix A of this report for abstracts of the papers and see *Workshop Proceedings on Strategies to Protect the Health of U.S. Deployed Forces: Assessing Health Risks to Deployed U.S. Forces* (NRC 1999c) for the full papers.

It is planned that in 2000 an NRC committee will review this report in conjunction with its sister reports, and a comprehensive analysis will be provided to DOD.

What Is Not Covered in the Framework

This report is not itself a risk assessment but only a proposed framework within which such assessments can usefully be conducted. No attempt has been made to carry out actual assessments of risks.

The report also does not attempt to describe or review established risk-assessment practices; it is not a treatise on the methodologies of risk assessment, a critique of their adequacy, or a prescription for their extension and reform. The field of risk assessment has spent much of the last 20 years debating the challenges to available methods, including extrapolation of animal responses at experimental doses to humans at environmental exposure levels and the ability to accurately describe human exposure levels. Controversies about the ability of risk analysts to provide accurate estimates of exposures and consequent risks, and the difficulties of fully accounting for the complexities and uncertainties in the underlying determinants of these exposures and risks, will continue to exist, and the present report cannot solve them.

This is not to say that the issues do not bear discussion, exploration, and, most especially, examination for their particular role in the assessment of risks to deployed forces. Several of the most important issues are explored in more detail in the set of papers commissioned for this project rather than in the presentation of the framework itself.

Furthermore, although exposures and experiences outside of the deployment context are clearly of concern to the larger question of health and safety protection, this report focuses on the sources of hazard specifically associated with deployment. Moreover, although general categories of threats are discussed and appropriate approaches to assessing them explored, no attempt has been made to create and maintain a comprehensive catalogue of threats that need to be assessed.

This report also does not constitute a review of the current DOD system. Partly by necessity, but mostly by design, the risk-assessment framework proposed in this report is a comprehensive general approach to the problems of assessing sources of threats to the health and safety of deployed troops, unconstrained by reference to particular practices and programs, including those that already exist as part of DOD's current efforts in this arena. Accordingly, omission of reference to existing programs and lack of analysis of how they might fulfill the objectives set out in the framework should not be taken to imply criticism of those programs or judgments about their value.

DOD has in place a wide variety of programs and activities for identifying threats, assessing potential exposures and risks, setting exposure standards, and designing equipment, operating procedures, doctrine, and training to manage risk effectively. Ongoing industrial hygiene procedures are carried out, including sampling and monitoring of exposures. The extensive military health care system tracks the health status of personnel. Collectively, this large set of activities and the planning that ties the components together could be thought of as comprising the current system in place at DOD for the protection of the health and safety of troops. Although an attempt has been made to acknowledge these activities, there is no attempt to catalogue the activities that are in place or systematically assess their effectiveness, either as individual elements with their particular goals or collectively as a comprehensive system of troop health protection. To do otherwise would require a much more extensive and systematic review of existing practices and programs than would be possible within the current scope and resources of this project and would demand a different array of expertise among the investigators. Similarly, many DOD activities fall under the regulatory authority of various federal regulatory agencies, and the role of such regulation in the arena of health protection of deployed troops is not specifically examined.

Finally, although a good deal of time was spent debating the question of psychological stress as a threat itself, the lack of established ways to assess the risks of such stress was acknowledged. Rather than try to address this issue in the framework proposed here, or to commission a paper on the matter, it was decided to note this as an important but unstudied area that will need broad, continuous attention by DOD. This omission is a shortcoming of the framework, since psychological stress is an issue of major importance to the health of deployed forces and deployment veterans, and any solution to how DOD should approach disorders and unexplained symptoms among veterans must include consideration of the contribution of stress. Further work on this issue is recommended.

ORGANIZATION OF THE REPORT

This report consists of five chapters. Chapter 2 discusses the factors and trends that should be considered in assessing risk to deployed forces and presents objectives for a deployment health-protection program. Chapter 3 examines existing frameworks for assessing risk and their utility for developing a framework for deployed forces; in addition, special aspects that are relevant to risk analysis for deployed troops are discussed. Chapter 4 describes a proposed framework for assessing risks to deployed forces, and Chapter 5 presents recommendations for strengthening and implementing the framework.

2

Rationale and Objectives for Examining Risks to Deployed Forces

A number of factors and trends were examined to determine what the military can and should do to protect the health and safety of deployed forces. These include factors relating to the nature of the deployment environment, the degree and nature of nontactical and tactical threats, including increased threats from chemical and biological warfare agents, changes in the nature of deployment and warfare, and the increasing responsibility that the military is expected to take in examining and protecting against the health and safety risks of its troops. This chapter attempts to review some of these factors and recommends objectives that should be considered in designing a program for the protection of the health of deployed forces.

DEPLOYMENT ENVIRONMENT

Deployment of forces in hostile or unfamiliar environments is inherently risky. In the garrison, the environment is chosen to be well protected, well known, and well controlled, and the activities of garrisoned personnel follow familiar practices that can be designed with a high premium on safety. In contrast, the deployment environment is, in large measure, imposed by the military mission. Each deployment can display a novel array of military and nonmilitary threats, known and unknown, with mission objectives dictating that these be dealt with as they come. Many activities carried out in this environment are not routine; tasks must be accomplished with the means at hand, despite potential dangers, in a setting where time, materiel, and attention are at a premium and where excessive precautions might engender their own risks or jeopardize the military mission. In short, during deployment, threats to the health and safety of troops might be multiplied or magnified, while the means to ameliorate or avoid them might be circumscribed.

DEGREE AND NATURE OF THE THREAT

The roles of U.S. military forces are changing and expanding. The world is becoming more multipolar, yet the United States has emerged as its principal military power. Increasingly, U.S. troops are deployed for operations other than war, including a variety of peacekeeping, humanitarian, and nation-building missions of varying scope and duration. Accordingly, deployments differ markedly in the degree and nature of tactical risk (i.e., risk due to the presence of an enemy or adversary). U.S. forces must be prepared for a spectrum of direct opposition, from essentially no opposition to various degrees of political opposition, civil unrest, thuggery and lawlessness, terrorism, insurgency, and low- or high-intensity combat.

With or without such tactical threats, however, there are risks of accidents, disease, and ill health that might be attributable to deployment. These might arise from contaminated local environments, from the intensive activities of the deployed forces, from exposures to hazards associated with mission tasks from such intentional exposures as use of pesticides and prophylactic agents, and from the rigors of exposure to climatic extremes. Troops might also be under considerable psychological stress owing to separation from family and familiar settings. This might be complicated by fatigue and a rapid operational tempo in which every task has heightened importance yet reduced margins for completion and error. Troops in hostile settings also have an understandable concern about their personal safety, and might show adverse effects from the stress of contemplating potential dangers and uncertainty about what the future might hold.

CHEMICAL AND BIOLOGICAL WARFARE AGENTS

Although most major military powers, including the United States, have formally renounced development and maintenance of chemical and biological warfare capabilities, the relatively modest technological challenges and costs for producing such agents has led to increasing concern about proliferation to rogue states and terrorist groups. As with all weapons of mass destruction, even when unused, the credible threat of their use can give considerable leverage, even against a superior force. The very isolation, economic pressure, and overwhelming military power with which the world community attempts to contain embattled and desperate factions might tempt them to seek influence through the leverage that chemical and biological weapons appear to provide. Despite the irrationality of using such weapons, the mere possibility of using them results in the deployment of expensive and cumbersome countermeasures and prompts caution about engaging such an adversary in any way that might expose large numbers of troops or civilians to a possibility of attack.

CHANGING NATURE OF DEPLOYMENT AND WARFARE

Large advances in technological capabilities, the shifting spectrum of missions, and the evolving nature of military threats have led to pronounced changes in the nature of deployment and of warfare itself. (See Appendix A.) Deployment of U.S. ground forces is increasingly characterized by an array of smaller, highly mobile units coordinated by a technically sophisticated communications system. Technology is also the key to the systems that give such units great capabilities for detection of tactical threats, direction of fire, and rapidly updated information about the state of the battlefield. There is an ever-developing ability to carry out remote sensing and real-time environmental monitoring for agents that might pose health threats. These current and emerging capabilities, and the flexibility and rapid response they enable, are critical to the military effectiveness of modern force deployment. (See NRC 1999a for a detailed assessment.)

To be effective, this strategy depends on the smooth functioning of its technological basis. To maintain flexibility and mobility, operational overhead must be limited as much as possible. Yet to maintain operational independence, each unit must be equipped with the means to detect and respond to threats—including environmental monitoring and sensing technology—and must bear the logistic burden of the equipment's transportation, operation, and maintenance, as well as the risks of its failure. Smaller, more-specialized units lead to lower redundancy of special skills and specialties, and loss of key personnel can put whole units at increased risk. Moreover, individual units can become somewhat isolated from central support and supply services, including medical services. There is a tension, therefore, between the provision of means to detect, protect against, and treat the consequences of exposures to potentially harmful agents in the deployment environment and the burdens this places on the units that must carry them out.

Three major changes stand out in the nature of deployment. First, increasing numbers of women are deployed, including missions of a widening variety of hazards. Analyses that might in the past have concentrated on male vulnerabilities and physiology will have to be broadened in scope. Second, the use of reserves in deployment situations is becoming increasingly frequent. Reserve troops have a different and more diverse set of experiences than regular forces, and the opportunity to use records of their recent activities or to prepare them for protection against threats might be circumscribed. Third, there is a pronounced trend toward operations in conjunction with allies, raising concerns about coordination of practices and the ability to form and adhere to standard operating procedures that allow planning and command structures to have the flexibility to accommodate harmonization with forces of other nations.

CHANGING EXPECTATIONS AND ESTABLISHING TRUST

The increasing technological sophistication of modern U.S. weaponry, both offensive and defensive, and the growing gap between U.S. and other forces, has created a remarkable ability of U.S. and allied forces to deliver destructive force with pinpoint accuracy while troops are deployed in relative safety far from the immediate zone of engagement. In recent engagements, air supremacy has been readily achieved, and the combination of such dominance, stealth technology, and precisely guided munitions has led to the perception that overwhelming military force can be brought to bear on an adversary with minimal risk of U.S. casualties, with reduced risks of casualties and collateral damage among the adversaries. A notion has developed that, at least in some military situations, one can employ "surgical" strikes and to a degree achieve "clean" warfare without undue and unnecessary carnage and destruction. Despite recent successes (albeit qualified ones) in this regard, there are clear limits to this ability, chiefly when the control of territory demands the use of ground troops and close engagement. Nevertheless, expectations about the ability of U.S. forces to avoid significant casualties have markedly increased in recent years, both in the military itself and in the minds of the general public and its governmental representatives.

This expectation of safety for deployed troops extends to risks of nonbattle casualties. It applies particularly to the variety of missions for operations other than war, in which tactical risks are much reduced and there is less of a public perception that troops are being put in harm's way. This increasing expectation of low risk from noncombat military service can be seen as part of a larger social trend in which large institutions, perceived as having power over people's lives, are increasingly held responsible for any impact on the safety and well-being of those who might come under their influence. This notion of responsibility has come to include matters that were once deemed unavoidable hazards of life or matters in which people were expected to look out for their own safety. Concomitantly, there has been a progressive erosion in recent years in the public's trust that large institutions will indeed attend to the needs of individuals rather than sacrificing them to institutional ends.

This distrust of large institutions affects the discourse about environmental protection and public health among the public, governmental regulatory authorities, and industry. In particular, public concerns about exposures to low levels of environmental contaminants are affected precisely because of the difficulty of establishing (or refuting) causal pathways on health effects suffered by individual citizens; many of the concerns are for health effects with multiple and complex causal pathways that might be well separated in space and time from the appearance of indicators of ill health. The associations between exposure and disease are statistical and the analyses are conducted on whole populations, but individual instances of tumors, birth defects, and autoimmune diseases are rarely directly attributable to particular causes or separable from the "spontaneous" cases of such health effects. The institutions that conduct the population-level analyses, if mistrusted, might be seen as using the ambiguity to dodge or misdirect responsibility for individual cases.

A deeper discussion of the issues surrounding risk communication and the public trust in risk assessment and management can be found in recent reports of national blue-ribbon panels: *Understanding Risk: Informing Decisions in a Democratic Society* (NRC 1996) and the two-volume 1997 report of the Presidential/Congressional Commission on Risk Assessment and Risk Management, *Framework for Environmental Health Risk Management*, and *Risk Assessment and Risk Management in Regulatory Decision-Making* (PCCRARM 1997a,b).

Although these factors have been discussed in the setting of civilian environmental protection, they also affect perceptions of the military's execution of its responsibilities for the health and safety of its troops, perhaps all the more so because of the degree of control the military exerts over the actions and exposures of its personnel, its need for secrecy in many matters, and its need to call for individual sacrifice for the sake of the institutional mission and the national interest.

Establishing and maintaining trust in such situations requires demonstrable diligence and success in several areas: (1) acknowledging and actively addressing responsibilities for the welfare of those under one's influence; (2) exhibiting competence, objectivity, and thoroughness in recognizing, investigating, and analyzing potential threats; (3) implementing forthright communication of risks to those subject to them; and (4) establishing a history and reputation of doing all these things openly, consistently, and well. This includes acknowledging past failures and taking appropriate responsibility for consequences. Owing to the causal ambiguity mentioned above, technical blame for specific health outcomes is often difficult to establish, but responsibility can be shown by taking a

constructive role in finding public solutions to public health problems, even controversial ones, rather than seeking mere technical absolution.

The military must seek to establish trust in its program to attend to the health and safety of troops in the face of some public questioning prompted by some recent controversies, including the exposure of troops to radiation from early atmospheric testing of nuclear weapons, the controversy over health effects among Vietnam veterans exposed to the herbicide Agent Orange, and the ongoing debate about illnesses reported by Gulf War veterans. These matters have been much studied and debated, and no stand is taken here on either the underlying scientific questions or the actions of the military establishment. What is clear, however, is that these controversies have been exacerbated by instances where military institutions did not fully take the opportunity to be proactive about potential dangers from exposures during military activities, to collect appropriate data before, during, or after these exposures, or to manage the aftermath in a way that bolsters public confidence that the military establishment is meeting its institutional responsibilities.

NEED FOR OPENNESS

The public expects the military to accept increasing levels of responsibility for all aspects of the health and safety of troops, while having that responsibility executed in public view. With the increasing interest in the environmental causes of disease, especially chronic disease, with the increasingly broad availability of scientific information, and with the burgeoning ability of interested parties to exchange information, trade concerns, and organize themselves using the internet, all decisions regarding health and safety are subject to considerable independent scrutiny.

More important, there is considerable scope for retrospective criticism and post hoc construction of hypothetical links between emerging symptoms or syndromes and past exposures resulting from deployment of forces, especially in view of the latency inherent between exposures and subsequent manifestations of chronic health effects. To the degree that potential threats, or questions about potential threats, have not been anticipated, it is difficult either to support or refute post hoc hypotheses, because the necessary information about toxic properties, interactions, and exposures is generally lacking.

OBJECTIVES FOR A PROGRAM OF ASSESSING RISK TO DEPLOYED FORCES

A central precept of public health is that prevention is preferable to treatment, and so emphasis should be put on prior recognition and characterization of potential threats. It is impossible, however, to examine every possible exposure scenario for every possible level of every agent in every conceivable combination. A program is therefore necessary to set priorities to determine which potential risk issues should receive more intense scrutiny, analysis, and/or data-collection efforts. This program should aim not only at characterizing known threats, but also at identifying exposures for which the threat potential is inadequately established. Such a program must acknowledge that certain hazards will nonetheless go unrecognized and that other hazards will not be altogether avoidable, although risky exposures might be reduced.

Thus, a program of vigilance for the emergence of unanticipated hazards during deployment is needed to supplement monitoring for detection and characterization of known threats and their impacts. Finally, personnel conducting ongoing and retrospective surveillance of troops' (and veterans') health status must be alert for effects that arise despite efforts at protection; these effects should be used to provide lessons for reducing risks in future deployments.

The exercise of assessing risk to deployed forces is not simply technical; it necessarily includes an analysis of the military's responsibilities—what it has a duty to find out about, and what it might later be held accountable for doing or failing to do. The critical goal of the DOD program to protect the health of deployed U.S. forces should be to articulate and fulfill these responsibilities. The technical procedures for doing so (the focus of this report) are merely a means to this end. For the program to succeed, these procedures must be executed competently and efficiently. But simply carrying out the technical tasks, however well this might be done, will not achieve the overarching goal. The results must be thoughtfully and vigorously applied to the achievement of the articulated objectives and the fulfillment of the military's responsibilities for the health and safety of its troops.

The program should have the following specific goals:

- to minimize the impact of disease and non-battle injuries;
- to develop a system to address risks and to execute the program efficiently;
- to establish DOD's reputation as willing to forthrightly address health and safety issues;
- to integrate risk awareness and the appropriate weighing of risks and benefits into decision-making, thereby eliminating unnecessary risk and controlling, or at least recognizing and understanding, those risks that cannot be eliminated, and ensuring informed decision-making concerning potential impacts on the health and safety of troops in the short- and long-term;

- to establish that the U.S. military is prepared to detect and to defend against threats;
- to characterize risks that might have arisen due to past exposures;
- to conduct present actions to minimize the degree to which they can be questioned in retrospect; and
- to do all the above without undue burden of cost or effect on military capability and effectiveness.

A unique aspect of risk assessment for deployed troops is the degree to which it might be necessary for commanders to weigh tradeoffs between risks to the military mission and risks to the health and well-being of the troops under their command. Questions regarding how such tradeoffs should be made and how much peril the troops should be subjected to in fulfillment of military objectives are key, but they are also beyond the scope of this report.

SUMMARY AND CONCLUSIONS

A number of factors and trends were evaluated to determine what the military can and should do protect the health and safety of deployed forces. The growing gap in capabilities between the U.S. and other nations or groups allows the possibility, and prompts the expectation, that deployment of U.S. troops even in hostile situations can entail risks that are far below historical levels. At the same time, the increasing threat from chemical and biological weapons with its looming possibility of significant casualties is changing the spectrum of tactical threats against which protection is required. Changes in missions and increasing use of U.S. forces around the globe in operations other than war focuses attention on threats of disease and non-battle injuries that differ from the concerns of avoidance and treatment of combat casualties. There is increasing recognition of the role of physical and psychological stress in prompting physiological changes that might have health consequences on their own or through interaction with other agents.

At the same time, the military is expected to take increasing responsibility for examining the potential health and safety risks to its troops, and the spectrum of concerns is broadening from acute illness and injury as a result of disease exposures, mishaps, and accidents to possible influences of low-level chemical and physical exposures on chronic diseases that might manifest themselves years later, perhaps long after cessation of military service. Some well-publicized cases have raised questions about both the military's procedures for identifying potential hazards before they manifest themselves, and in its collection of the information on toxicity, exposure, and health-status surveillance necessary to detect and monitor threats to the health and welfare of troops.

In view of all of these trends and changes, an examination of the military's program for the protection of health and safety of deployed troops is in order. There is a need for a process that is open and encourages scrutiny of DOD actions and the incorporation of health and safety concerns into all aspects of decision-making. Emphasis should be placed on the prior recognition of potential threats, and characterizing and setting priorities for them; monitoring for detection and characterization of known threats and their impacts; and ongoing and retrospective surveillance of troops' (and veterans') health status for effects that arise despite protective efforts. Such a system must acknowledge the military's responsibility for the health and safety of its troops.

3

Existing Frameworks and Special Considerations

Risk assessment has been used and methods developed over what now amounts to decades of practice in the fields of environmental health, occupational health, and engineering. The framework, structure, and policy-making for such assessments have been extensively examined, notably in a series of reports published by the National Research Council (NRC). The seminal report, *Risk Assessment in the Federal Government: Managing the Process,* widely known as the "Red Book" (NRC 1983), brought structure to the risk-assessment process and defined its key components in a framework that has been nearly universally accepted ever since. Key methodological issues were considered in *Issues in Risk Assessment* (NRC 1993a); the role of uncertainty and its analysis was further explored in *Science and Judgment in Risk Assessment* (NRC 1994); use of risk information by decision-makers and the public was considered in *Understanding Risk: Informed Decisions in a Democratic Society* (NRC 1996); and a series of reports from the Committee on the Biological Effects of Ionizing Radiation (the BEIR Reports) (NRC 1972, 1974, 1980, 1988, 1990, 1999d) has treated methodological issues for radiation risk. Regulatory agencies have promulgated guidelines and procedures for their conduct and application of risk assessment, notably the Environmental Protection Agency's (EPA's) guidelines and its more recent revision proposals (EPA 1996). These broad-level statements are supplemented by a myriad of documents detailing policies, procedures, and guidance for various specific applications. Variation in methodology among federal agencies and an analysis of how methods are influenced by regulatory mandates have been reviewed (Rhomberg 1997). Many more reports and treatises could be cited.

In short, the questions of how to frame such inquiries, how to approach risk-assessment tasks, how to handle problematic issues, and how to bring the results to bear on the motivating policy issues are well explored. This is not to say that all questions are answered—if they were, the ongoing flow of advisory reports would cease—but the issues that remain do so because of their inherent difficulty, rather than any lack of attention.

This chapter examines current general frameworks for assessing risk and their utility for developing a framework for assessing risks to deployed U.S. forces. In addition, special aspects that are relevant to risk assessment for deployed troops are discussed.

EXISTING FRAMEWORKS FOR RISK ASSESSMENT

NRC's Red Book Paradigm

Overview

NRC (1983) provides a structure for conducting risk analysis that has served as the basis of virtually all discussion of the topic since it was proposed 16 years ago. Although this structure is familiar, it is so central to this task that it is worthwhile to recapitulate the main findings.

The NRC report advocated maintaining a distinction between risk assessment and risk management. Risk assessment was defined as the attempt to come to an objective characterization of the risks entailed by the process or agent in question among the population of interest. Risk management was defined as the process of using this information, along with information on the costs, feasibility, and effectiveness of various control measures and consideration of the interests and preferences, rights, and obligations of the parties involved, to arrive at decisions about what course of action to take regarding the existence of the risks. The aim of drawing the distinction is to allow a legitimate place for economic and social values, the balancing of conflicting interests, and other extra-scientific considerations to enter the decision-making process, while avoiding the contamination of the characterization of risks by these considerations.

This prescription is frequently misread to suggest that risk assessment must consider only "best" or "central" estimates of uncertain risks and that risk assessment and risk management must be entirely separate exercises carried out by different analysts. In fact, too rigid a separation only serves to hamper communication of the risk information to the risk-management decision-makers, who are best served when they are informed about what is known, what is not known, what is likely, and what is less likely yet possible about uncertain risks. Some decisions might be sensitive to uncertainty in the risk estimates and others might not be; in some decisions, risk aversion has a role whereas others might require risk neutrality. In other words, risk assessment must be conducted so as to summarize what is known in an objective way, and to provide answers to the questions asked by the risk management process. These questions are quite legitimately value-laden, but the answers should aim at objectivity.

The technical and objective aspects of risk assessment must supply risk management with information that is technical, rational, and objective. In fact, the analysis of costs and effectiveness of alternative risk control or mitigation options is highly technical. Moreover, a large body of quantitative analytical methodology, usually referred to under the rubrics of operations research and decision science, can be brought to bear to find optimal solutions to allocating resources, by balancing risks against one another and against costs of mitigation, and to improve the design of procedures and actions that must be taken in the face of risk and uncertainty. These methods take as their inputs the characterization of risk provided by risk assessment and the characterization of the relative desirability of different outcomes, willingness to bear risks for certain ends, and willingness to expend resources to lower risks—factors that together comprise the values referred to above.

The full exploration of the analytical framework for risk management is beyond the scope of this report. But the spirit of this report's recommendation that the risk assessment framework be constructed to serve the ends of risk management requires careful attention to the kinds of analysis that risk information is intended to illuminate.

Returning to the Red Book's framework for risk analysis, the NRC (1983) proposed dividing the risk assessment-phase into four key components:

- Hazard identification—the assessment of the qualitative properties of an agent's toxicity, including an assessment of the weight of evidence that it might in principle be able to produce toxic effects in the population of interest, provided doses are sufficient.
- Dose-response analysis—the assessment of the quantitative relations between different degrees of exposure and the probability, magnitude, or severity of response to be expected among individuals in the target population.
- Exposure assessment—the estimation of the magnitudes of exposure or dose actually or potentially experienced by members of the target population in the situations of interest, including information on the variation in magnitude of this exposure in different circumstances.
- Risk characterization—in which the results of the other three components are brought together to provide estimates of the potential

impacts on the exposed population. Risk characterization also reviews the basis of the estimation and examines the contribution of uncertainties in the constituent elements on the uncertainty in the estimates.

The last step, risk characterization, is the point at which the analysis is condensed to the basic key findings that are likely to be most relevant to the risk-management process. It forms the interface between the two realms and can be thought of as belonging in part to each. The key for the risk assessor is to express findings that are most useful in risk-management decision-making. For risk managers, the key is to frame questions in a manner that best allows the technical analysis to bear on them.

Application of the Paradigm to Deployed Forces

Given the prominent role of the NRC (1983) paradigm in structuring risk analysis, how should it enter the present attempt to create a framework for the protection of deployed U.S. forces? First, although the paradigm was developed to assess toxic effects from environmental or occupational exposure to chemical agents, it is readily adaptable to analysis of a variety of hazards. This makes it appropriate to the protection of deployed forces, which face a variety of threats that must be considered in a common framework.

Hazard identification, for instance, can comprise any analysis of the qualitative properties of a threat to deployed forces. Although the specific means of inference will differ, the central concept of hazard identification applies equally well whether the threat is the possible carcinogenicity of an industrial chemical, possible mechanical failure of a complex piece of machinery, possible disease caused by a poorly understood infectious microbe indigenous to a remote deployment site, possible use of a certain military tactic by an adversary, or the impacts of physical or psychological stress on the troops' morale and fighting effectiveness. The common conceptual elements of hazard identification include (1) determination of the nature of impacts to be sought; (2) determination of the hazard's potential mode or modes of action; (3) description of losses or adverse outcomes that might be caused by the hazard; and (4) assessment of the basis for the present understanding of these properties (based on past experience, analogy with similar threats, experiments, or expert judgment) and our confidence that the properties so discerned apply to the particular setting. The result of this analysis is an assessment of the likelihood that specific adverse outcomes will be caused by specified conditions of exposure.

Similarly, the concept of exposure assessment can be applied to the attempt to measure or estimate any quantities that express the varying degree or intensity of encounter with the source of threat, whether it is the uptake of a chemical from the environment, number of duty cycles for a machine, or concentrations of microbes in drinking water. The aim of exposure assessment is to examine the specific instances in which the undesirable outcomes are risked. This is achieved by defining and measuring quantities that describe the setting-specific magnitude of encounter with the threat in such a way that the probabilities of manifestation of the adverse outcomes are functions of the exposure magnitude. That is, the dose measurement is the independent variable, and the dose-response function is the expression of how the probability or magnitude of response is thought to vary as a function of the dose (Rhomberg 1995).

The NRC (1983) four-step paradigm for risk assessment allows a diversity of threats to be examined in a common context. It is recommended that even those types of hazards that are not usually explicitly analyzed using this paradigm be so analyzed by using it in the framework for assessment of risks to deployed forces. For example, risks of combat casualties, traffic accidents, aircraft malfunctions, industrial accidents, terrorist attacks, disease outbreaks, and adverse weather conditions could all be analyzed under a paradigm of similar conceptual structure. This would facilitate integration of the results of hazard-specific assessments and tracking of the complex process of simultaneous consideration of multiple threats, a critical part of organizing relevant information and developing risk management strategies, including trade-offs.

The NRC (1983) paradigm, however, is not sufficient by itself as a risk-assessment framework for protecting deployed U.S. forces. Although the paradigm can be applied to a variety of threats, it is constructed on the premise that one has already identified the specific hazards to be assessed and the settings in which exposure is expected to occur. That is, the NRC (1983) paradigm is a strategy for exploration, analysis, and characterization of particular threat scenarios that have previously been recognized and defined. It does not deal with the process of recognizing which particular actions and practices in a complex process (such as troop deployment) might require analysis of specific threats. It provides for no systematic way to catalog such threats, to set priorities for them, or to prepare a characterization of how the spectrum of hazards might change between deployments or locations, or as a particular deployment continues. It focuses on characterizing specified exposure scenarios rather than discovering modes of exposure or assessing the likelihood of circumstances that might lead to encounters with hazards.

In short, the standard structure of the NRC (1983) paradigm is a key part of the needed structure, but it should be nested inside the larger context of a comprehensive analysis of and response to the spectrum of potential impacts on the health and safety of deployed troops and on mission success. To a large measure, the framework proposed herein is constructed to address these needs for an overarching structure.

A full risk-assessment framework for deployed forces needs to address these issues as a way of identifying hazardous situations and resulting exposure scenarios, which can then be examined and more fully characterized in the context of the traditional NRC (1983) paradigm. Moreover, the framework needs to provide for integration of the results of such analyses into a larger risk-management process in a way that tracks the completeness of the analysis and facilitates bringing the results to bear on achievement of the program's objectives. A framework proposed by the Presidential/Congressional Commission on Risk Assessment and Risk Management (PCCRARM 1997a,b) aims at considering this larger structure. It calls for embedding the risk analysis steps inside of a risk management decision-making context. The process is described as having six steps.

The first step is to characterize the risk management problem, including the goals of the process, the nature of the relevant data, the decision-making structures that will be applied, the roles of stakeholders, and the means of involving them. The second step is the risk analysis per se, conducted using appropriate methods while keeping in mind the questions the process is aimed at answering. The third step is the analysis of options to control or ameliorate the risks, with consideration of how actions on one risk will affect others and the costs and benefits of various actions. By explicitly placing the analysis of options in the framework, the ability of the risk analysis to make the distinctions necessary for choosing among options is highlighted. The fourth step is to make decisions based on the information on risks, goals, and expected consequences of various options, as determined by previous analysis. The basis of the decision should follow from the criteria set up at the outset. The fifth step is to take the risk management actions decided upon, and the sixth is to evaluate the effectiveness of those decisions, checking to see if the intended results indeed occur, and feeding the experience into improvement of the process in further iterations of the cycle.

This is a structure for both risk assessment and risk management, and, thus, it goes beyond the strict scope of what is being attempted by the present framework, which focuses on the characterization of risks. The Presidential/Congressional Commission's design has an important lesson, however: the risk assessment process must bear in mind the questions being asked of it by the larger risk management, decision-making process in order to identify the distinctions that need to be made in choosing courses of action, the ways in which risk assessment results should be expressed so as to be useful in making decisions, and the way in which risks interact with one another and with the costs of addressing them.

Another important lesson is that stated goals are necessary, and the success of the process at achieving those goals should be subject to ongoing evaluation. The framework developed in the present report attempts to embody the spirit of the Commission's approach. While it does not take on the full problem of risk management for deployed forces, it does attempt to examine some of the aspects of that management that are particular to the context of deployed forces health protection and the consequent demands that this puts on the risk assessment process.

Another existing framework to consider is the one applied in environmental public health surveillance (Weeks 1991; NCEH 1996; Thacker et al. 1996). The primary issue here is to achieve public health protection by detecting the existence of threats as they are happening through programs of surveillance. Once detected, further evaluation can determine causal pathways and opportunities for prevention and intervention. Depending on the nature of the threats, it might be more efficient to conduct surveillance for hazards, for exposures, or for outcomes. Tracking outcomes in the population of interest has the advantage of detecting the impacts and might be appropriate when causes are unclear or when effects can result from multiple causes, but the disadvantage is that adverse impacts must happen in order to be detected. If causes cannot be established, opportunities for prevention might be circumscribed. Once particular exposures are recognized as potentially harmful, conducting surveillance for instances of such exposure provides the opportunity for intervention before undue harm is caused. Surveillance for hazards, if possible, is preferred in that it gives the earliest opportunity to intervene, preventing exposures before they begin.

This public health surveillance approach is applicable to the situation of troop deployments. In the framework developed herein, outcomes surveillance largely correspond to the recommendations for health surveillance during and after deployments. Companion reports examine health surveillance issues (IOM 1999) and exposure surveillance (NRC 1999a). To a large degree, the emphasis of the framework suggested in the present report is an attempt to embody the aims of hazard surveillance, and the lesson learned from the public health paradigm is the need to seek out unrecognized potential sources of harmful exposure.

The Kaplan-Garrick Definition of Risk

Overview

Another seminal publication that addresses the structure of risk analysis and contributes to the approach suggested here is the first paper to be published in the journal *Risk Analysis*, a treatise on the definition of risk by Kaplan and Garrick (1981). Risks in their definition are sets of triples, each formed by (1) a scenario (i.e., a hypothetical future event or set of events), (2) the likelihood of the scenario occurring, and (3) the consequences of the scenario. A risk question can be expressed as a mutually exclusive set of such triples, with each set determined by selecting alternative courses of events, and each set having its own probability of transpiring and probable outcome.

This definition calls attention to some important facts about risks. For one thing, risk is about uncertainty and indeterminacy. In doing risk analysis, there is no need to be sure in the prediction of outcomes, only a need to express a belief regarding the likelihood of the different possible outcomes. The point of the risk analysis is to characterize the probabilities as a guide to what actions should be taken now in the face of an uncertain future course of events.

There is sometimes confusion about this aspect, particularly in risk assessment of environmental contaminants, because the problem is cast as one of predicting what will happen to the health of people who happen to receive a certain dose of the agent. When, owing to lack of information or incomplete understanding of the underlying biology, this prediction is subject to great uncertainty, it is sometimes said that one "cannot do risk assessment" because the risks are too uncertain. In fact, this confuses two aspects of risk analysis. One aspect is the attempt by the analyst to use information and scientific understanding to narrow, insofar as possible, the uncertainties about the consequences of exposure and the probabilities of the consequences occurring. It is ironic that, to the extent that the analysis succeeds in being able to make such predictions with certainty, it ceases to become a risk analysis in the strict sense because there is no longer uncertainty about any adverse outcomes. The second aspect of risk assessment is to acknowledge and characterize the uncertainty that remains, and to communicate that characterization as input in an analysis of what should be done in the face of that uncertainty.

Even when predictions can be improved, they rarely can predict which particular individuals in an exposed population will succumb to an adverse health event. At the level of the exposed population, one might be fairly confident in predicting, for example, the approximate fraction of people who will become ill after ingesting water contaminated with an infectious microbe, but for each exposed individual the risk is whether or not he will be among that fraction.

This illustrates that, in characterizing a risk, the way in which the possible courses of events are divided into distinct scenarios depends on the question being asked. In the example just mentioned, a population-level analysis might define the set of scenarios as "no one in the unit becomes ill," "a few troops in the unit become ill," or "a substantial fraction of the unit becomes ill." At the individual level, the scenarios might be "I do not become ill," "I become slightly ill," or "I become seriously ill."

The Kaplan-Garrick definition of risk also points out that the probabilities involved are Bayesian probabilities, in that they are best guesses about of the likelihood of the alternative courses of events. As further information is gained, these probabilities can be updated to reflect a more thorough understanding. The uncertainty arises both because outcomes are contingent on the unknown course of future events and because of the limits to understanding the causal processes involved.

Application of the Definition to Deployed Forces

The scope of the risk analysis dictates how the alternative scenarios are defined. In practice, because there might be many possible unfoldings of events that are of interest, the set of scenarios can become very complex. Often, scenarios are not single events but rather compound sets of events, some of which might be more easily analyzed as separate components of the overall risk. For example, in analyzing the potential benefit of providing protective garments to troops deployed in a region where terrorists might sabotage chemical storage facilities, the threat to the troops' health (the outcome of interest) occurs as a result of a complex scenario. For analysis, one might divide the compound event into a series of components, perhaps including the likelihood that troops will be stationed near such a storage facility, the likelihood that it is indeed sabotaged, the likelihood that the released chemical plume is transported in the direction of the troops, the likelihood that warning devices will operate correctly, the likelihood that troops will nonetheless get a critical level of exposure, and the likelihood that individual soldiers will succumb. Very different kinds of data, modeling, and analytical approaches are needed to estimate each of the probabilities in this chain. The best route to estimating the likelihood of the whole scenario is to separately analyze the parts, allowing for the contingencies. Moreover, analyzing chains of events in this way permits greater insight into how probabilities of end consequences change in a real situation as the actual course of events unfolds. In addition, scenario analysis provides focus on the points where actions and equipment operation have their effects on risks, providing targets for risk management strategies. It also calls attention to junctures where different risks can interact. In the example just discussed, the protective garments may cause their own impacts on health and well-being or they might exacerbate reactions to other agents.

In general, components that are valuable to analyze are (1) the likelihood of the presence of a hazard associated with a deployment; (2) the likelihood of releases of agents into the environment, given their presence; (3) the likelihood that troops will suffer exposure (of various magnitudes), given the releases; and (4) the likelihood that health effects will be caused among them, given the exposure. Clearly, the specific way in which complex scenarios are broken down will depend on the particular instance, but components like the ones just suggested might often be involved. The value of looking at whole scenarios is that it emphasizes that threats must be dealt with in context, not one by one, with attention to the ranges of exposure as well as the toxic properties of agents that might be encountered. It parses the problem into parts that can be addressed by different kinds of analyses, and identifies components that take different amounts of effort and data collection to address. Assessing how various activities and practices affect the safety and health of deployed forces should involve tracing the consequences of alternative deployment practices and activities through their effects on exposure and possible adverse outcomes, bearing in mind the likelihoods of the various components. For instance, in the chemical storage sabotage scenario discussed above, the benefits of protective garments can be analyzed in the context of the likelihood that their protection will come to be needed compared to the decrement in military performance and troops' well-being that their use might entail. The opportunity for interaction of prophylactic agents and procedures with other hazards can be noted and the need to understand such interactions pointed out.

This view of risk analysis is somewhat more expansive than is often taken, but it serves the purposes of a framework for assessing threats to deployed forces. A more traditional approach might begin by focusing on identified toxic agents, then assessing their potencies, identifying likely exposure scenarios and characterizing their consequences, and then investigating what changes in practice might avoid or mitigate the risks. What such an approach tends to lack is a focus on finding those aspects of the whole body of activities and practices that might entail some sort of hazard. In quantitative assessment of risks to deployed forces, the likelihood that exposure events will come to pass might be as, or more, important than the probability of adverse effects to a given exposure.

SPECIAL CONSIDERATIONS ABOUT RISK ASSESSMENT FOR DEPLOYMENT

It is worthwhile to ask what special considerations are required for a framework for risk analysis in the case of assessing threats to the health and safety of deployed troops. Some of the special challenges and needs surrounding risk analysis for deployed forces are discussed in Chapter 2. Here, we examine how the practice of risk analysis might need to be adapted to meet those needs. Several technical matters suggest some alterations in conventional risk-assessment methodology and other issues that relate to the unique risk-management challenges presented by troop deployment—challenges that the framework for conducting analyses of threats to deployed forces should be designed to address. Because risk analysis is above all a practical discipline, aimed at addressing the questions at hand, it is well to review the special considerations for deployed-forces risk-assessments.

Need for a Comprehensive Catalog of Hazards

The military is in need of a comprehensive catalog of assessments of all of the hazards that actually impinge or might impinge on deployed troops, and not just a threat-by-threat analysis. Many troops might be exposed to many of the relevant threats simultaneously, and their protection entails addressing the whole array of threats. Any action taken to address one threat is likely to alter the risks from other threats. This means that the incremental, piecemeal approach that a regulatory agency might take in addressing the various hazards under its purview might not by itself be sufficient. This approach places a great premium on cataloging all of the potential threats and setting priorities for them for detailed attention, but it still requires a framework for operating on many fronts at once. The primary objective is the integrated analysis of the spectrum of threats that troops might experience. Moreover, the question "Threats to whom?" has diverse answers: one is interested in threats to the health of individual service personnel while deployed, in cumulative career-long and life-long risk profiles, and in threats to the capabilities of whole military units or to the success of missions.

DOD Is a Regulator and Is Regulated

DOD has roles akin to being both the "regulating" and the "regulated" parties in many of its risk-assessment activities in the sense that it must identify hazards and establish health-protection exposure criteria on the one hand and act to implement those criteria on the other. (It is also true that many risk-assessment activities fall under the authority of other governmental regulatory bodies.) Although some assessment is carried out as an internal risk-management process, the effectiveness of this process is subject to external criticism and expectations. In the world of environmental regulation, the division among regulators, the regulated community, and interest groups in a publicly debated give-and-take process plays a role in shaping approaches to health-protection measures and in ensuring scrutiny and review of results. This interaction needs to be replaced by an alternative review process in the military setting.

The Military Mission Has Primacy

When considering acceptable risks, the needs of the military mission must receive primacy. Although the challenge of risk trade-offs is universal, it plays a particularly marked role in the military setting. With sufficient military justification, it might be necessary to accept more risk than would be possible in a civilian setting. Accommodations for safety have consequences on military effectiveness and risks to the mission, personnel, and materiel that might be immediate and potentially large. Although risks of immediate casualties have always played a large role in military planning, the attention paid to possible longer-term chronic effects with delayed impact is a newer and increasing concern. This entails explicit recognition of the necessary trade-offs that are made between military effectiveness, mobility, and preparedness, on the one hand, and risks of immediate casualties, longer-term loss of health and well-being of service personnel, potential future governmental liabilities for treatment and compensation of deployed veterans, and even effects on morale and the reputation of the military for protecting troops, on the other hand. The burdens produced by accommodation of health and safety concerns, comprising equipment, logistic impediments, and training, as well as time and attention, can affect the military significantly. One must also consider risks induced by prophylaxis and protective equipment in balance with the risks from hazards they are designed to combat.

Margins of Safety

Because of the foregoing, incorporating "margins of safety" or conservative estimates of acceptable exposures, as is frequently done in environmental and occupational health settings, is not always useful to the needs of military risk management. When a high level of health and safety protection can be achieved without undue burdens or increases in other risks, such margins can be part of an effective risk-management program. But when risks must be borne or when probabilities of casualties must be weighed against immediate military considerations, best estimates of probable impact are more useful. The proper use and interpretation of uncertainty factors is complex and a full discussion is beyond the scope of this report. Risk assessment best serves risk managers when there is a careful distinction among needed extrapolation adjustments, allowances for uncertainty, and out-and-out margins of safety. Whether assessments for deployed troops need special values for the uncertainty factors is a question worthy of further consideration.

Utility to Field Commanders

During deployment, especially in high-intensity situations, consequential decisions affecting responses to or defense against potential hazards might often need to be made by field-level commanders with modest relevant technical expertise and little time to gather and analyze relevant data. In civilian environmental health decision-making, in which issues are usually less pressing, it is typically possible to more thoroughly analyze specific situations, accumulate and analyze data, and subject the questions to centralized expert analysis. In the military situation, however, there is a great premium on anticipatory analysis and contingency planning so that sufficient information and careful, expert analysis can be used to prepare insight into difficult situations before they occur. There is also a need for designing operational procedures for use during deployment that capture the key considerations of risk-management problems. These procedures would provide straightforward guides and tools for commanders, allowing them flexibility and freedom to make rapid yet appropriate decisions based on changing current situations without abandoning the larger health and safety considerations.

Intentionally Created Hazards

Environmental hazards might be insidious, but they do not arise from malice. In contrast, troops can be subject to intentionally created hazards through terrorism or sabotage, and these hazards can be aimed specifically at the troops' vulnerabilities.

Different Types of Risk

The specific nature of many of the threats to troops is different from threats that are encountered in the civilian risk-assessment setting. There are no well-established methods for assessing risks for some potential threats of particular importance to deployed troops, such as from infectious diseases or from psychological and physical stress.

Specialized Exposure Conditions

Many exposure factors are different for deployed troops, and the standard assumptions made for general population environmental protection or for industrial hygiene applications might need modification for the military setting. Deployment durations (and hence, exposure durations) can be less than the career-long or lifelong assumptions usually made, but work days could be longer (up to continuous), inhalation rates and water consumption higher, opportunities for dermal contact increased, and modifications by climate might be important. Food and water sources can be controlled or at least partly controlled.

Multiple Exposures

Troops during deployment could become exposed to a number of threats simultaneously. Exposures that are individually tolerable without appreciable risk might not be so when several are experienced together, and the question of interactions among agents looms particularly large for deployment risk assessment.

The Population at Risk

The nature of the population at risk in the military setting is different from the civilian setting. Compared with the general population, troops are typically young and healthy (and perhaps more tolerant of threats), yet their exposure in settings of high physical or psychological stress might raise susceptibility. As a group, they are as racially and ethnically diverse as the general population, so susceptibility variation due to genetic differences is not reduced, but it might be possible to develop and use information on individual genetic susceptibilities to limit exposures to those who suffer the most risk. Most troops are young when exposed; they will have more time than the general population for the effects of long latency to appear, and such effects will be less subject to diminution by competing risks. Young troops have most or all of their childbearing years ahead of them, and female troops face the possibility of deployment during critical but perhaps unrecognized early stages of pregnancy. Exposures during deployment, and any after-effects they might produce, can be potential factors in the health status of the troops through a long life. Whether these special features of the population at risk warrant alteration of traditional uncertainty factors or inclusion of special quantitative considerations is a question worthy of examination.

DOD's Control Over Population at Risk

The military has a considerable degree of control over the population at risk and its actions regarding that population. This gives opportunities to modify or control exposures in ways not available in a civilian setting, and it also requires that a degree of responsibility be taken for the appropriateness of actions and risks imposed on troops. The military has the potential to gather and utilize a good deal of information about locations of troops, their activities, their exposures, personal medical and exposure histories, genetic differences, and characterization of baseline rates of exposure—all information not readily available to civilian risk managers. There is the potential to make assignments based on past exposures or special sensitivities, avoiding exposures of those particularly susceptible to a hazard. The availability of this information and the ability to exert a good deal of control over the locations and activities of its personnel leads to opportunities and challenges. One can entertain an approach in which control of activities around sources of risk or tracking of cumulative exposures is used to ensure that individuals do not exceed a quota of risk. Although this approach is used for radiation workers, it is considered inappropriate for most civilian occupational settings. In contrast, civilian environmental regulators must assume that the population acts as free agents, so it is necessary to control sources of exposure rather than to control the actions of the public in encountering those sources.

DOD's Special Responsibility in Managing Risk

Because much of military activity entails higher risks than are typically found in general civilian life, because almost every command decision at all levels is to some degree a decision to expose someone to more or less of those risks, and because military personnel have, in the interests of organizational efficiency, discipline, and the common good, ceded some of their personal control over their lives and actions to this command structure, the military has a particular responsibility to manage risk-taking wisely and fairly. The military also has the need to call for individual sacrifice, acting to put its troops at hazard of life, limb, and health in the interests of the nation at large. This setting poses special challenges for risk management and for risk communication with the affected population. Articulating these responsibilities is beyond the scope of this report; it is not a risk assessment task per se, but it should affect the priorities and foci of DOD's risk assessment efforts. It is part of the process of using risk analysis to fulfill the public's expectations about the military's stewardship of the health and well-being of its personnel.

SUMMARY AND CONCLUSIONS

Previous examinations of the framework, structure, and policy-making for risk assessments provide useful information for developing a risk assessment framework for deployed U.S. forces. One of the most important and relevant outcomes of those efforts is to conduct risk assessments so as to provide useful answers to the questions asked by risk managers.

The NRC (1983) paradigm for risk assessment has maintained a prominent role for structuring risk analyses in ways that are useful to risk managers, and the paradigm is readily adaptable to deployed-forces protection. However, it does not deal with the process of recognizing what particular actions and practices that are done in a complex process (such as troop deployment) might lead to threats that need to be analyzed. That need is fulfilled by incorporating the Kaplan and Garrick (1981) definition of risk into the NRC (1983) paradigm. From that basis, a risk-assessment framework can be developed with components to analyze: (1) the likelihood of the presence of a hazard associated with a deployment; (2) the likelihood of releases of agents into the environment, given their presence; (3) the likelihood that troops will suffer exposure (of various magnitudes), given the releases; and (4) the likelihood that health effects will be caused among them, given the exposure. Such a framework begins by examining *activities* rather than *specific agents*, as is done in more-traditional risk assessments. In that way, efforts would be focused on how activities and practices come to present threats, how likely it is that threats will be manifested in practice, and how mitigating one risk might raise other risks.

In addition to drawing upon existing risk-assessment frameworks, it is important to consider special needs and aspects of U.S. troop deployment. A useful framework in this context must be aware of DOD's need to accomplish inherently risky missions while also protecting its troops from a wide variety of hazards that can be caused unintentionally or intentionally. Also, the framework must be responsive to DOD's need to make risk trade-off decisions. Therefore, risk estimates must be realistic (not overly conservative) and readily useful to field commanders. In addition, the uncommon exposure conditions and types of hazards encountered during deployment, as well as troop population characteristics, warrant special consideration.

4

A Framework for Assessing Risk to Deployed Forces

The proposed framework for risk assessment of threats to deployed U.S. forces is intended to organize risk-assessment activities. It is divided into several components, providing places for various analyses, and organized to illustrate the role of each activity and how it contributes to an overall analysis of risks to deployed forces. The object is to foster a systematic approach to recognizing and cataloging potential hazards, founded on examination of the various activities and settings of deployment. Each recognized scenario or sequences of events that could lead to potentially hazardous exposures is divided into components for analysis, and these analyses can then be applied in judging the likelihood that potentially hazardous exposures will indeed be encountered and, if encountered, the probabilities that adverse outcomes will be engendered. This information can then be used to consider modifications of procedures, equipment, and actions to avoid or mitigate risks with the awareness that actions taken with respect to one risk might affect others and might need to be weighed against the needs of the military mission.

The framework puts great emphasis on recognition of potentially hazardous activities, including systematic processes to uncover previously unrecognized ones. It also emphasizes anticipatory analysis and contingency planning before actual deployment as a means for identifying preventive measures and allowing risks to be carefully analyzed before they actually arise. Finally, it provides for the collection of appropriate data before, during, and after actual deployments.

The framework is characterized by three major enterprises—ongoing strategic baseline preparation and planning, specific deployment activities, and post-deployment activities. These enterprises are characterized by separate modes of activity and analysis, but are connected to each other by their common application to achieving the goal of assessing risks to deployed forces and by their need to incorporate each other's results. The elements of the three enterprises are presented in Boxes 1, 2, and 3, and how these elements fit in the overall framework is illustrated in the form of a hierarchical tree diagram in Figures 1 to 6. Although a single tree encompasses the whole framework, owing to its complexity, it is necessary to represent the tree in a series of diagrams to indicate how the subparts are connected. Figure 1 presents the three major enterprises of the framework, Figures 2 to 4 depict the activities encompassed by the ongoing strategic planning enterprise, Figure 5 outlines activities to be undertaken during deployment, and Figure 6 illustrates the post-deployment enterprise. This chapter explains and elaborates upon each of the risk-assessment activities of the framework.

ONGOING STRATEGIC BASELINE PREPARATION AND PLANNING

Ongoing strategic baseline planning comprises all of the activities and analyses concerned with preparation, through analysis, systematic investigation, risk-aware design of procedures and materiel, and contingency planning for threatening eventualities before they occur. As such it includes all activities concerned with recognizing potential threats, anticipating the circumstances under which they might arise, and assessing and characterizing each kind of threat qualitatively and quantitatively. The aim is to make a thorough examination of the processes, activities, and settings that might arise during deployment, to identify potential hazards (including previously unrecognized hazards), and to subject them to appropriate analyses. Although the present report does not explore risk management in depth, the ongoing preparations also include preventive measures such as setting exposure standards and modifying procedures to avoid or ameliorate risks. The activities are not tied to specific deployments, but represent the continuing development of information about potential deployment risks and exposures, organized through the framework so as to create an ever expanding and improving base of knowledge. This knowledge can be drawn on to increase the capability to avoid or mitigate risk and to refine doctrine and training so as to lead to safer deployments. That is, the first phase comprises ongoing, long-term activities aimed at increasing preparedness for risk mitigation issues in specific future deployments, since planning and preparation for specific deployments (which fall under a second, subsequent phase of activity, described below) must often be conducted at an accelerated pace.

BOX 1
Ongoing Strategic Baseline Preparation and Planning Activities

Identify Potential Threats
- Lists of known and suspected agents
  - Battle injuries
  - Chemicals, radiation
  - Disease
  - Stress
  - Accidents
- Exposure
  - High, intense
  - Unusual, novel
  - Persistent, cumulative
- Inventories of exposure associated with activities and settings
  - Hazards associated with deployment per se
    —specific environments
  - Hazards associated with missions (by type)
    —combat
    —operations other than war
  - Hazards associated with places (by place)
    —terrain, climate, infrastructure
    —indigenous diseases
    —local environmental pollution
    —toxic industrial chemicals
    —adversaries
- Co-exposure pattern review

Develop Priorities for Detailed Analysis
- Likely to occur
- Mission-critical
- Known threat
- Potential impact
- Special DOD responsibility

Risk Analysis
- Probability of release
- Probability of exposure given release
- Probability of health effect given exposure
  —hazard identification
  —dose-response
  —risk characterization
- Recognition
- Environmental consequences

Incorporation into Standards and Risk-Aware Planning (Risk Management)
- Design, doctrine
- Standards development
  —operational
  —emergency/crisis
  —cumulative
- Contingency plans
- Training
- Review

BOX 2
Specific-Deployment Activities

Deployment-Specific Planning
- Update with mission-specific information
- "Before" biomarker samples

Upon Arrival
- Surveillance sampling

During Deployment
- Recognition of events and detection of exposures
  —detection

During Deployment (continued)
  —concentration
  —concentration × time profile
- Vigilance for unsuspected exposures
- Sampling, archiving, record-keeping
  —biological samples
  —environmental samples
  —unit activities, positions
  —monitoring and detection activities

Deployment-Termination Activities
- "After" biomarker samples

BOX 3
Post-Deployment Activities

Reintegration
- Post-deployment service
- Veterans

Data Archiving
- Capture during-deployment data
- Implement deployment-specific follow-up systems

Ongoing Health Surveillance
- Individual examinations tied to deployment history
- Implement registries with triggers for deeper analysis

Population Analyses of Associations
- Exposure reconstruction
- Epidemiological analyses
- Generate hypotheses and test with new toxicological studies

Evaluate Lessons Learned
- Deeper understanding of known threats
- Study previously unanticipated threats
- Feedback to predeployment planning mode

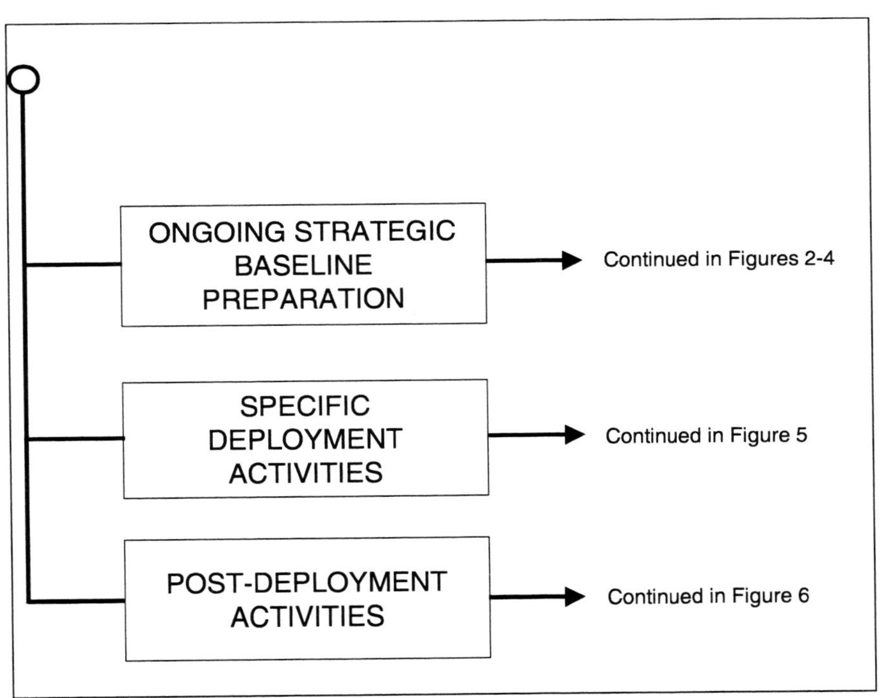

FIGURE 1. The three enterprises of the proposed risk-assessment framework.

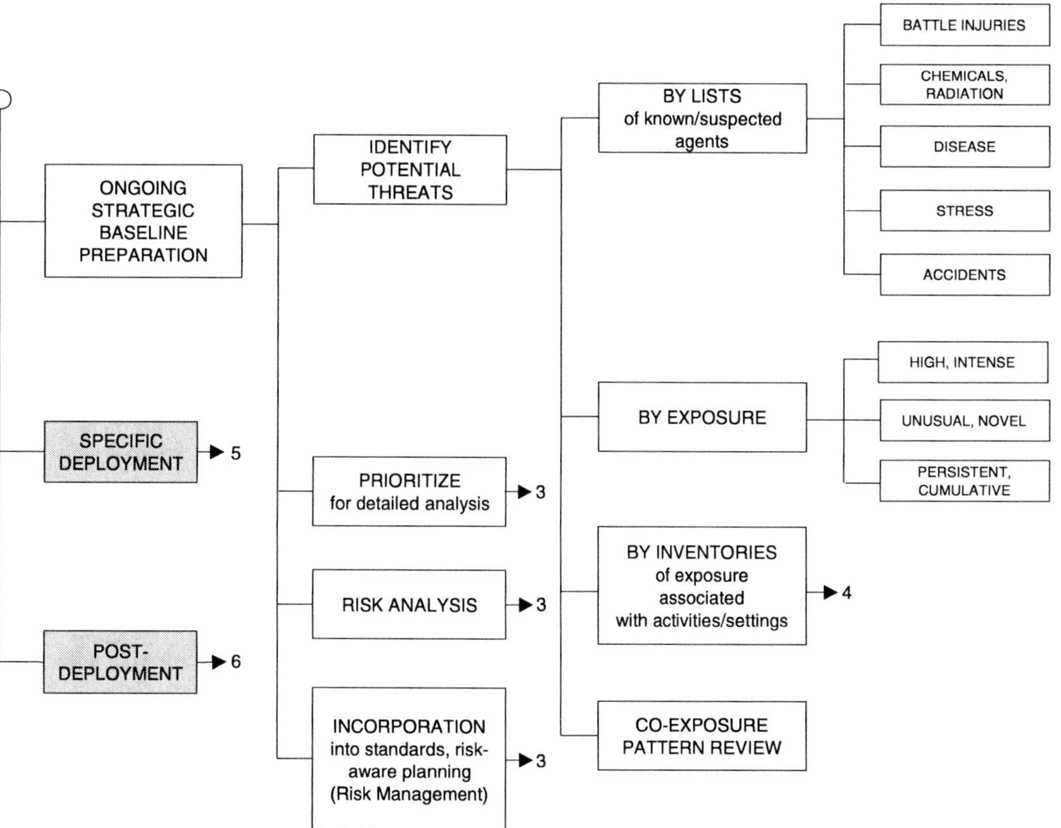

FIGURE 2. Ongoing strategic baseline preparation. The numbers correspond to the figures, which provide more detail about the activity.

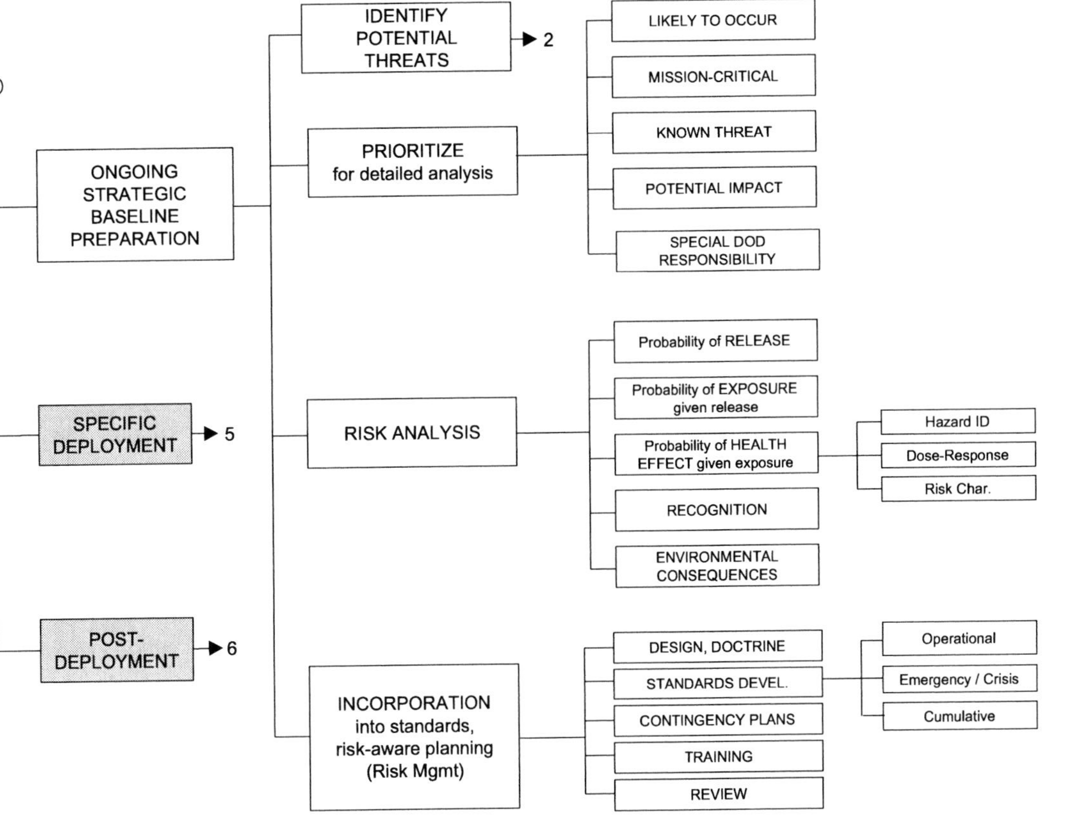

FIGURE 3. Ongoing strategic baseline preparation (continued from Figure 2). The numbers correspond to the figures, which provide more detail about the activity.

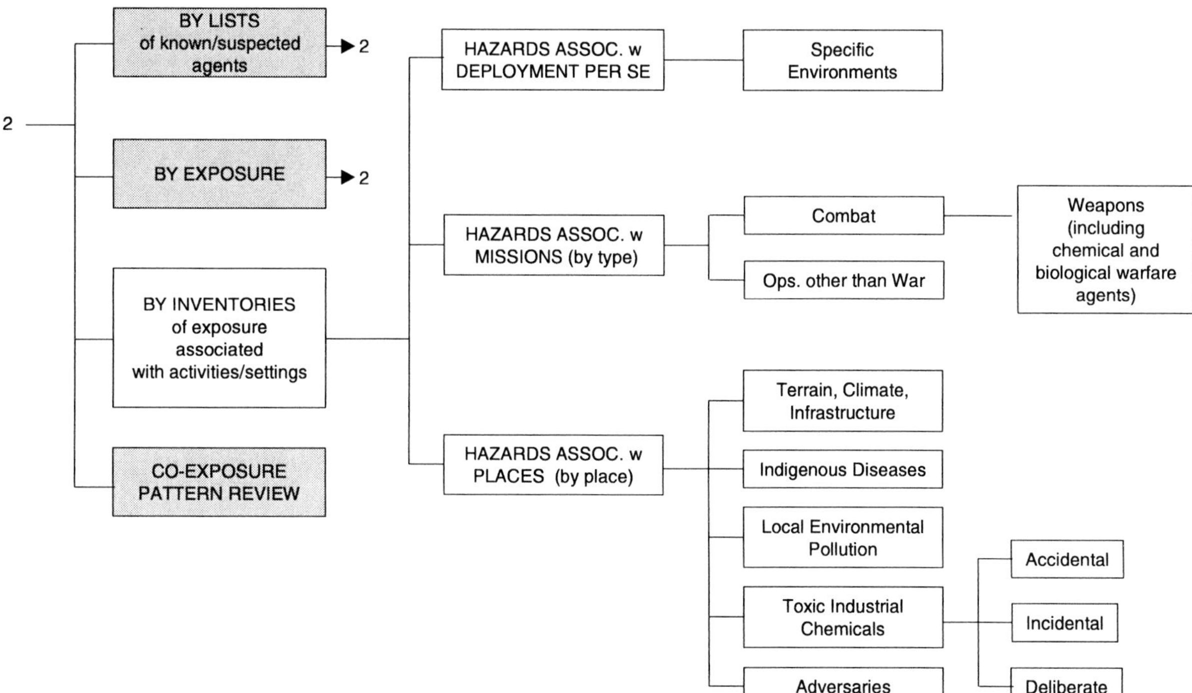

FIGURE 4. Ongoing strategic baseline preparation (continued from Figure 2). The numbers correspond to the figures, which provide more detail about the activity.

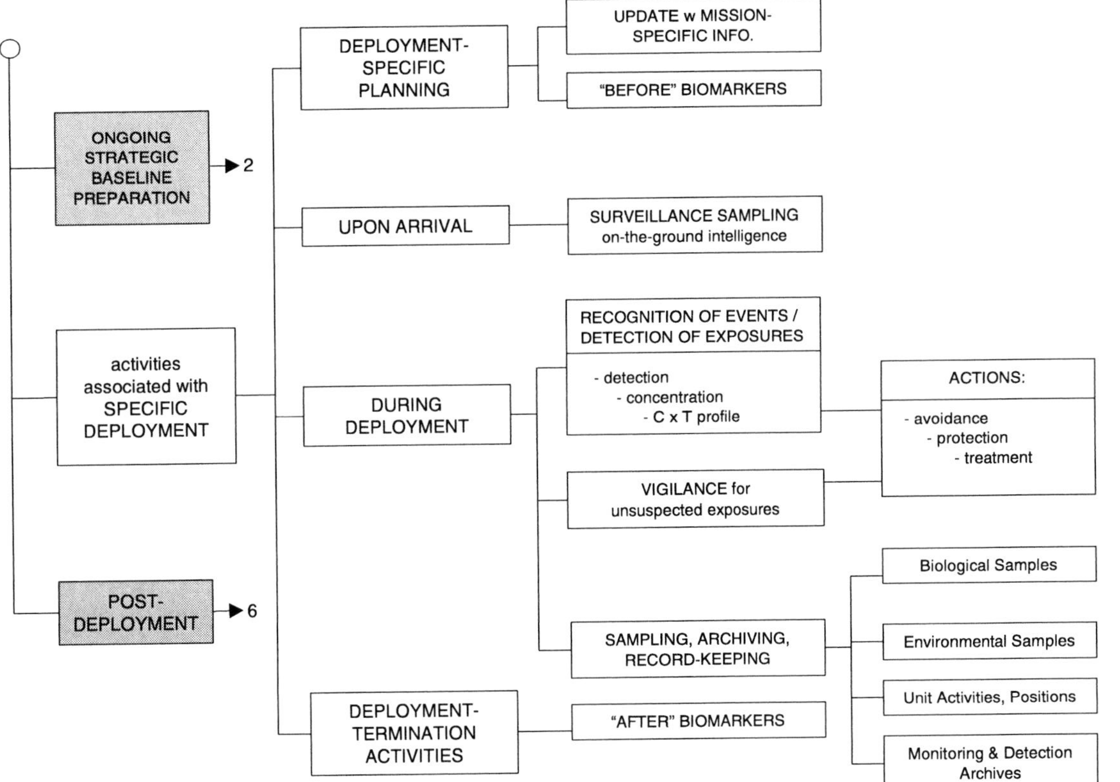

FIGURE 5. Specific deployment activities. The numbers correspond to the figures, which provide more detail about the activity.

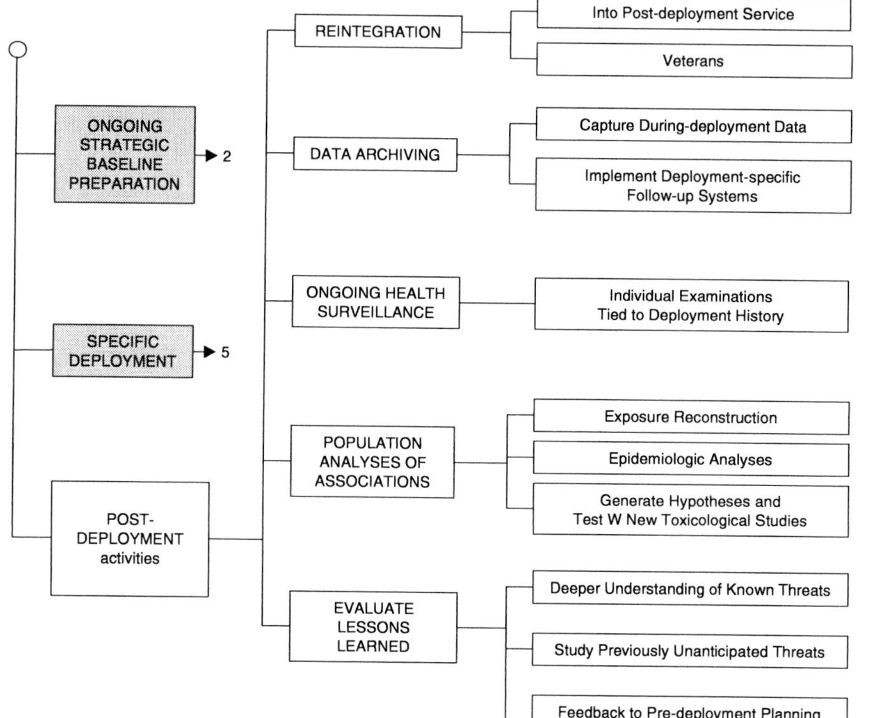

FIGURE 6. Post-deployment activities. The numbers correspond to the figures, which provide more detail about the activity.

This phase of analysis is clearly large and complex, containing many distinct components of activity (Figures 2 to 4). It is divided into four major steps: (1) identify potential threats; (2) develop priorities for detailed analysis; (3) conduct a risk analysis; and (4) incorporate understanding of risk into standards and risk-aware planning (i.e., risk management).

Identify Potential Threats

The first step is to identify potential threats, both the agents of harm and the circumstances, activities, and settings that might cause potential threats to be realized. The aim is to systematically sort through activities to identify potential sources of hazard, including ones that might not have been recognized in this setting, or at all. Unrecognized threats could include agents not previously listed as hazards or new properties of recognized hazardous agents (such as chronic toxicity from ongoing low-level exposure). Clearly, the task of sorting through the whole universe of deployment-associated activities and settings is daunting, and the call to identify all potential hazards, including novel ones, is idealistic in view of the scarcity of data that usually prevails. In practice, a series of screening exercises, described below, can be pursued. The point of setting such a challenging goal is to go beyond a focus on agents already on standard lists of hazardous agents and activities, or on the most obvious properties of those agents.

This step is different from the traditional process of hazard identification, which focuses on marshaling and interpreting the evidence regarding the toxic potential of particular agents considered individually. It is also different from the usual process of identifying a list of potential agents of concern (as one might do in evaluating a toxic waste site), because it seeks to identify hazards rather than simply recognize potential exposure to a list of known hazards. Unlike a toxic waste site, where the exposures are there to be measured, the task here is to imagine potential exposure scenarios and the likelihood that they will occur during deployment. What needs to be examined is not just the agents and exposures, but the activities and settings that lead to exposures.

The practical means that is recommended for pursuing this search for hazards is to conduct several different screening exercises in parallel, each based on a somewhat different rationale. The intent is that by approaching the common question from several different angles simultaneously, one increases the probability that situations in which potentially harmful exposures might arise are recognized as such. Examples of such approaches are to screen (1) by lists of known or suspected hazardous agents; (2) by exposure considerations; (3) by inventories of exposures associated with various activities or settings; and finally (4) by conducting a review of the hazards identified by the previous three methods. This last approach is used to identify likely patterns of co-exposure among agents that should be given special attention due to the possibility of accumulative or synergistic effects.

Lists of Known or Suspected Agents

Notwithstanding the advice not to rely solely on established lists of hazardous agents, it is wise to begin by consulting such lists for presence of agents associated with deployment tasks. Established sources of characterization of hazards could be consulted for several different kinds of threats, including battle injuries, chemicals and radiation, disease, physical and psychological stress, and accidents. A paper commissioned by the National Research Council (NRC) for this project (Rose 1999; abstracted in Appendix A), lists many infectious diseases that should be considered.

In addition to the Department of Defense's (DOD's) own existing lists, hazardous agents can be sought from such sources as the U.S. Environmental Protection Agency (EPA) Integrated Risk Information System and Acute Emergency Guideline Levels for Hazardous Substances, the Agency for Toxic Substances and Disease Registry Toxicological Profiles, the Hazardous Substance Data Base, the American Conference of Governmental Industrial Hygienists documentation, the International Agency for Research on Cancer monographs, EPA Health Effects Assessment Summary Tables, the National Toxicology Program Annual Report on Carcinogens, and the State of California Proposition 65 list.

The review of such lists should go beyond the properties that caused the agents to be listed, because listing might be prompted by the most sensitive among several toxicity end points or by a particularly prominent toxicity end point. The hazards that an agent might pose during deployment might be affected by likely exposure patterns that differ from those considered in the original listing. Similarly, the presence of an agent on some list of toxic compounds is not a substitute for full hazard identification. The object of this initial step is to recognize potential hazards for fuller consideration in the risk-analysis step.

Exposure

A second means of seeking potential hazards is to examine agents with notable exposure patterns. The aim of this process is to identify agents to which deployed troops are likely to be exposed, putting a premium on the need to understand their potential hazardousness. The thinking here is similar to that applied to the current discussion about testing of high-production-volume chemicals (Environmental Defense Fund 1997). In this process, agents call attention to themselves through particularly high or intense exposures in the deployment setting; exposures that are unique to the deployment setting (or at least are unusual elsewhere); through exposures to new compounds (such as prophylatic medicines or combustion products of innovative materials); or through exposures to persistent compounds or those that might accumulate in the body. For agents with such exposure patterns, there is a high premium on DOD's ability to address the potential for toxicity, and if sufficient data are lacking, a high priority for appropriate testing is indicated. Although most agents that receive attention due to notable exposure patterns might end up not being particularly hazardous, establishing that this is the case is an important part of attending to the possibilities of threats to the health of deployed troops.

Inventories of Exposures Associated with Deployment Activities and Settings

Under this approach, the main focus is on examining activities and settings for the exposures and the potential risks they entail. As such, it represents the greatest departure from the usual approach of beginning with agents and exposures and then examining the activities where potential hazards arise. In this task, methods can be borrowed from the disciplines of life-cycle impact analysis and pollution prevention (Curran 1996; Barnthouse et al. 1997; Pojasek 1998; NAE 1998). The method entails systematic review of the activities that occur during deployment, and for each one, considering what exposures it entails, what materials it consumes, what waste products it emits, what products it produces, where the inputs will come from, where the outputs will go to, and the accidents and failures that might occur. The outputs of some processes might become the inputs of others. The point is not simply to scan or examine activities for known or obvious hazards, but to use the exercise to prompt consideration of what might be hazardous and what investigation is needed to understand its safety and risks.

This process serves several purposes. It constitutes an aid to recognizing potential hazards that might not otherwise be obvious. It highlights exposures to agents that are insufficiently understood and provides a basis for developing investigative priorities of such agents. It serves to link exposures to hazards directly to the activities that cause them, facilitating the development of risk-control measures, and it puts the development of such measures directly into consideration of the whole spectrum of threats that an activity could entail (and which might be affected by measures to control one of them). It also serves as a basis for linking events into scenarios for quantitative analysis of the likelihood that potential hazards will indeed lead to adverse impacts.

The application of this approach in the military situation should be particularly fruitful because, in contrast to most organizations, the military has already put a lot of thought and analysis into how it conducts its tasks. To organize the task of examining activities and to enhance the utility of such an analysis in planning particular deployments, it is useful to break the process into parts that focus on (1) activities associated with deployment per se, (2) activities related to type of mission, and (3) hazards associated with particular places.

Activities associated with deployment per se are those entailed in most deployments as a result of needs for transportation and the provision of food, water, and shelter, as well as those associated with widely used equipment. These activities would include use of pesticides and insect repellants, standard vaccinations, waste disposal, exposure to exhaust fumes, and exposures associated with the operation and maintenance of military equipment. In short, they cover all of the potential hazardous exposures that deployed forces bring with them wherever they go on whatever mission. It might be useful to further segregate this category into subcategories describing deployments to different classes of environments, such as warm or cold, wet or dry, urban or rural.

Activities associated with missions include those specific to the type of mission the deployed forces are sent to accomplish. Clearly, combat has its own distinct set of activities and hazards, and this could usefully be broken up into a number of subcategories. Threats from the use of chemical and biological weapons (including the hazards associated with protective measures against those weapons) could form its own subcategory. The wide variety of missions for operations other than war could be classified into categories of efforts that entail distinct sets of activities and exposures to potential hazards.

Hazards associated with places, the third category, comprise those threats that are indigenous to the places where troops are deployed. The key here is to develop information about hazards that might be encountered in different locations around the globe so that this information will be available if ever needed. Information should be gathered on climate, terrain and infrastructure, on industrial facilities and the materials used, on the degree of contamination of local environments, and on the identity of the contaminants. Especially important is the question of local endemic diseases, because many of these may be unfamiliar and poorly studied.

Hazards associated with places can be subcategorized into those attributable to (1) local terrain, climate, and infrastructure (bridges, dams, floodplains, and roadways); (2) indigenous diseases and vectors; (3) local environmental pollution; (4) toxic industrial chemicals; and (5) various adversaries that U.S. forces might face. The threat from toxic industrial chemicals (as distinct from local pollution) comes from the possible release of stored chemicals or supplies at industrial or depot sites. Such releases might be entirely accidental, occur incidentally as an unintended consequence of other activities (e.g., a storage tank being hit by an errant missile), or be released deliberately by sabotage or terrorism. Assessment of the variations in threats associated with adversaries relies on judgments about potential opponents' military capabilities, weaponry, and tactics.

Dividing the inventory of activities associated with deployment into components allows the development of a base of information that can be used quickly when a new deployment is anticipated. This inventory generally can be combined with that appropriate to the specific mission and that to the specific location of the deployment to yield a deployment-specific catalog of threats. This inventory also gives opportunities to note the ways in which particular hazards might vary in their importance in different specific deployments, for example, if several agents with similar mechanisms of toxic action might be expected to be experienced together in certain combinations of mission and location.

Co-exposure Pattern Review

Co-exposure pattern review constitutes an evaluation of the results of the previously discussed examinations of hazards, notable exposures, and inventories of activities. The review is used to identify instances in which simultaneous exposures to agents might be a result of several different activities, possibly leading to greater effects than if the various exposures were experienced separately. It will also identify cases of simultaneous exposure to different agents that might be suspected of acting synergistically. Determining which combinations of agents have the potential to interact in this way is a difficult challenge. The matter is discussed in much more detail in a paper commissioned by the NRC for this project (Yang 1999, abstracted in Appendix A). Agents that affect one another's pharmacokinetics, that act on similar target organs, or act by similar mechanisms of action are prime targets for such considerations. The aim of this review step is to identify those situations that should be subject to deeper scrutiny and perhaps toxicological experimentation (see Yang 1999).

Develop Priorities for Detailed Analysis

The inventory created in the step that identifies potential threats might be quite large, and a clear view of potential hazards might in many cases be hampered by lack of data. An exercise to develop priorities is therefore necessary to identify those situations most in need of further analysis and data collection. In addition, in cases in which the emergence of adverse effects follows from a complex chain of events, each of which requires analysis, it is necessary to decompose the scenario into its components, all the while assuring that all components in the chain receive sufficient attention so that the priority of the originating scenario is maintained. An example of an event in a complex chain that might require analysis would be a mechanical failure of a device leading to released chemicals in a wind-blown plume leading to contaminated vegetation through which troops may need to pass.

This step to develop priorities has similarities to the discipline of comparative risk analysis in that it seeks to compare a wide array of hazards and identify which ones have the greatest likelihood of occurring and the greatest potential impact, and therefore deserve priority attention. (It differs, however, in that one is developing priorities for potential hazards for further risk analysis rather than preparing risk estimates for regulatory attention.) There are several criteria that would suggest high priority:

- *Likely to Occur.* Those hazards most likely to be experienced in practice should be given high priority, all else being equal. Hazardous activities or events less likely to occur (but having consequences if they do) can receive lower priority, but need to be investigated in time, or else one runs the risk that the unlikely events transpire before an investigation has been done.
- *Mission-critical.* Hazards that could affect the chances of success of military missions must receive high priority for attention.
- *Known Threat.* If the potential impacts of a hazard are known, then scenarios involving exposure to that hazard, or unresolved questions about the circumstances that might lead to exposure, need to be investigated.
- *Potential Impact.* All else being equal, hazards with large potential impacts, including those that have effects beyond the immediate actual losses, should receive high priority. Low-probability, high-impact events can be given lower priority but should not be ignored simply because they are unlikely, because even the expected value of loss might be large. There is some obvious and unavoidable circularity in these criteria because one has to do some quantitative analysis of probabilities to know that a hazard is likely, critical, or large. The process of developing priorities must be based on extant or preliminary information, experience, and judgment. When priorities are sensitive to judgments or assumptions that might be questioned, obtaining information that can resolve such issues itself becomes a priority.

- *Special DOD Responsibility.* It is important to identify potential hazardous situations that DOD might be especially held responsible for investigating before allowing its troops to be exposed. It is difficult to define in general terms what those situations are, and attempting to do so is beyond the scope of this report, but instances can be recognized, mostly having to do with things that are not "supposed to be" risky, but that in fact might be. These situations include exposures that are special to military situations and not experienced by civilians, and situations in which the military exposes troops to agents with unknown properties for its own military mission. DOD should consider how its special responsibilities might be construed and how to apply this understanding to the question of investigating hazards.

The object of developing priorities is not to sort those hazards that will be investigated from those that will not be. DOD ultimately has responsibility for investigating all of the potential hazards. The point of developing priorities is to provide the military with a rational sequence of hazards to assess.

Data Limitations

Risk analysis must always contend with the challenges of limited data. Guidelines for action in the face of harmful impacts will always be needed, while the information on which to base such decisions will always be limited, leaving some uncertainty about the existence and magnitude of risk. From case to case this uncertainty might vary but will always be present, and its impact should be judged against the urgency of the decision the analysis is meant to inform and the gains or losses to be experienced under alternative courses of action. Risk analysis does not require certainty about the hazards it attempts to characterize; indeed, as argued in Chapter 3, risk analysis might best be viewed as an investigation into our uncertainty about what potential impacts might befall the subjects of the analysis. This uncertainty comes not only from the contingency of outcomes on unknown future events, but also from our incomplete understanding of the applicable causes and effects.

The present framework urges a very comprehensive approach to investigating potential threats to deployed forces; it advocates consideration of the whole spectrum of potential threats from diverse sources and it calls for attention to all potential health effects of agents, not just those causing the most notable effects or those calling attention to the agent as a hazard in the first place. This approach is necessary if one is to be proactive about recognizing potential hazards, but the wider this net is cast, the more data will be needed and the more instances will be encountered where attempts to characterize risks must be based on a very meager base of relevant information.

There are three areas in which data might be lacking. First, existing information might raise possibilities of adverse outcomes following exposure, but the data might be insufficient to provide robust answers about the magnitude or even the true existence of the risk in the population of interest. This leads to uncertainty in the characterization of tentatively recognized threats. Second, there might be insufficient data about actual levels of exposure or about the profiles of susceptibility of those exposed, leading to uncertain application of the understanding of the hazard in a particular instance of interest. Third, there might be adverse effects from an agent that are currently unrecognized because the agent has not been appropriately tested or because the existing tests are not sensitive enough or applicable to the human exposure settings of interest.

In facing the limitations of data, there are two pitfalls to be avoided. The first is to confine attention to those cases that are relatively data rich, on the grounds that more satisfactory, dependable answers can be obtained. This can result in overlooking important risks simply because they are have been overlooked previously. The second pitfall is to get bogged down in attempts to supply all the missing data, bringing all cases up to some ideal standard of information availability before seriously considering their risk analysis. Since resources are always limited, this quest can never be fulfilled.

Faced with many risks to consider, a paucity of data about them, and limited resources to gather new data and conduct the risk analyses, what is a responsible risk analyst to do? A two-pronged approach is necessary. First, risk analysis must be content to say what can be said and not only to acknowledge the inevitable remaining uncertainty, but to try to characterize that uncertainty so that appropriate perspectives on the meaning and robustness of the analysis are expressed. Historically, this approach has been stronger in some sub-fields of risk analysis than in others. It is an area of active methodological development, and DOD is advised to participate fully in this endeavor. Discussion of specific methods is beyond the scope of this report, but general accounts are available (Morgan and Henrion 1990). The general approach follows from the conception of risk articulated by Kaplan and Garrick, discussed in Chapter 3. The alternative possibilities for outcomes are laid out and their relative likelihoods are assessed in view of the data available—the better the data are able to narrow down the reasonable interpretations, the higher the likelihood associated with those outcomes and the lower the weight given to alternatives.

Characterization of uncertainty and the limitations of available data are important to all risk analysis, but they might play an especially important role in the analysis of deployment threats, where high-consequence decisions might require taking one risk to avoid others. Risk management approaches exist to help make such decisions, but when the risks to be compared are quite uncertain, or uncertain to different degrees, good characterizations of the uncertainty is necessary in order to arrive at sound solutions.

In addition to such characterization of uncertainty, the second prong of the approach is to reduce the uncertainty by gathering more data. Given the limitation of resources, only a small amount of new data will be obtainable, and thus prioritization is necessary. Among competing needs, the relative priority for obtaining data should depend on (1) the costs of not having the data (such as losses due to suboptimal actions in the face of the uncertain risk, e.g., undergoing significant costs to avoid an exposure that actually poses little risk or failing to take easy measures against an unrecognized risk); (2) the costs of obtaining the data; and (3) the likelihood that the data, if obtained, will help settle the outstanding issues or result in a sufficient reduction in uncertainty that it was worth obtaining the data. Methods to employ these principles in determining the benefit of additional data on a risk question are codified in the established quantitative discipline of Value of Information Analysis (Clemen 1990; von Winterfeldt and Edwards 1986), which is further discussed in the companion report on exposure (NRC 1999a). The methods readily consider the costs involved with the delay entailed in waiting for data to be developed, an aspect that is useful in the deployment context, where issues arising during actual operations might need rapid responses on a timescale in which some information (such as exposure information) might be obtainable sufficiently quickly, while other information (such as toxicity information) might not be.

The criteria for developing priorities for detailed analysis of threats acknowledge that the risks in need of analysis are many, the applicable data are few, and the abilities to obtain additional data are limited. The criteria provide a guide to how pressing the need for analysis is in one threat relative to another. To the degree that a threat has high priority, it is important to consider obtaining the data necessary to understand it. That is, the priority gives a rough measure of the cost of not having data, referred to above, and the approach of Value of Information Analysis can be used to determine allocation of limited resources for obtaining further information.

Experience also provides important information about hazards, their impacts, and the circumstances that lead to manifestations of health and safety risks. As risk assessments are conducted, insight is gained into the nature of key questions, and data needs might be suggested, which should feed back into the prioritization of research. Tracking of the health experience of personnel during and after deployments provides important information that needs to be captured and fed back into the risk assessment process. These matters are more fully discussed later in this report and in an accompanying report (IOM 1999).

Risk Analysis

Once hazards and the circumstances under which they arise are identified, the tools of risk assessment can be applied to characterize hazards and exposures, and to conduct quantitative estimates of risk. These results can then be incorporated into decision making, such as planning, design of doctrine and standards procedures, and training. The risk-analysis step constitutes the core of the framework proposed here.

The hazards of concern vary a great deal in their nature, and their analysis varies greatly in the information available with which to characterize them and in the methods that have been developed to carry out that characterization. Risk projections might be based on actuarial data of past observations or incidence rates (e.g., the number of road accidents per vehicle-mile traveled), analogy with familiar risks, experimental data, or expert judgment. The confidence in the risk analysis will vary with the degree to which the setting for which estimates are made resembles the settings that are the basis for projection.

This section notes some commonalities among risk-assessment methods for different kinds of threats and calls attention to some special aspects of assessing risks for the purposes of protection of deployed forces. These matters may affect both the analytic methods and outcomes of risk assessments.

The general approach outlined in the NRC paradigm for risk assessment (NRC 1983) can be applied, not only for toxicity of chemical agents, but also for microbial and physical hazards. This paradigm facilitates focusing on the nature of the adverse impacts of concern, determining the measurable features of particular settings that affect the probability and/or severity of various adverse outcomes, and expressing the best estimate of the magnitude of risk as a function of those measures of exposure to the hazard.

In certain cases, the potential for exposure is more important to assessing overall risk than the potential response to the exposure (Rodricks 1999). For example, a high rate of casualties is expected among unprotected troops immediately downwind of a major release of a volatile nerve agent. The exact level of impact depends on the degree of exposure and the responses of the exposed troops, but the principal driver is the likelihood that such a release indeed happens. The real larger question is what is the risk to troops "exposed" in the sense that they are present in a theater where weaponized nerve agent is present in the hands of an adversary. In this situation, the threat is not the nerve agent per se; instead, it is the course of events that leads to uptake of some small amount of the nerve agent. To address this larger risk question, one must assess the probability that the weapons are indeed used (contingent on the development of the conflict, assessed using military judgment and war-game simulations), the probability that they produce appreciable concentrations at the troops' location (contingent on winds and terrain and the locations of troops vis-à-vis the release point, assessed using fate and transport models), the probability that warning and protective measures fail (contingent on the performance of devices, equipment, and the troops themselves under duress, assessed using mechanical failure models, experiments, and training experience), and only finally (and least critical to the calculation, owing to its lack of case-by-case variation) the probability that an individual that takes up some agent succumbs to its toxic effects.

This view broadens the more typical exposure assessment procedures of exploring various modes of exposure and estimating variations in levels of uptake, by including the probabilities that the different exposure scenarios actually occur. The point here is that, for many situations of interest in protection of deployed troops, the likelihood that unfolding events might produce exposure might be of prime importance in assessing the overall magnitudes of risk.

The value of the Kaplan-Garrick definition of risk, discussed in Chapter 3, should be evident here. Beginning at a starting time and starting situation, one traces out the possible scenarios that describe the unfolding of future events, each scenario traced until its outcome of interest is reached. Because some scenarios require a chain of events to get to the outcome, the scenarios might represent compound events that might need to be broken up into a series of parts for analysis, each by appropriate methods. Often, it is useful to represent the unfolding of events in a tree diagram, with pathways of events splitting upon the occurrence of key events. The probability of each scenario transpiring (i.e., of each pathway down the tree) is estimated, and the probabilities for chains of events are estimated by finding the probabilities of their pieces, allowing for contingencies. The fact that the complex pathways are broken down into components for analysis does not alter the fact that the real risk questions are faced at the starting point of the analysis: What are the probabilities that the various end results will come to pass, and what impact will be suffered upon the arrival of each distinct possibility?

Structuring risk problems in this way is also valuable because it can clarify how risks change in actual situations as the events unfold, that is, as one proceeds down one branch of the event tree and not others. Continuing with the nerve agent example given above, once an agent-bearing shell explodes at a particular place, the issue of whether the weapon will be used is settled in the affirmative and the probability that a plume will move toward troops becomes highly case-specific, depending on the shell-burst site, the terrain, the troops' location, and the direction of the wind, all of which have the particular values for the current situation. This kind of analysis can be very valuable in planning responses to events, determining which properties of changing situations are key to the alteration of risks, and developing means to rapidly update generalized scenarios with situation-specific information. This information can then be plugged into the established analytical structure to give real-time risk information to commanders in the field.

Some of the key aspects to consider in risk analysis are the probability of release; the probability of exposure given release; the probability of a health effect given exposure; the probability of certain outcomes in specific deployment scenarios; and environmental consequences.

Probability of Release

The circumstances under which contained materials come to be released into the environment, and the likelihood of such releases, are frequently at issue. These are often approached using probabilistic fault-tree analysis to assess the chances of physical failures of the means of containment. The destructive forces of combat can greatly increase the probabilities of containment failures, even if the events are unintentional. To the extent that intentional human actions are involved in the releases (sabotage, terrorism, or use as weapons by adversaries), expert military judgment, experience, and the results of war games might have to be used.

Probability of Exposure Given Release

For agents that are released from specific places or at specific times, environmental fate modeling can be used to estimate the probability that releases lead to exposures of troops. Such modeling tends to be very dependent on local settings and conditions, however, because the various environmental components, the flows of media, and the impact of temperature, sunlight, and rainfall, can vary considerably. For agents that come to be well mixed into local air and water, or for local environmental pollution, the usual approaches for environmental contaminants can be used, in which the rates of consumption of air, food, and water are used to estimate ongoing intake rates of the contaminants they contain. The exposure factors that are used (inhalation rates, water consumption, body weights, exposure durations) should reflect the military situation, which might be different from the exposure factors used in civilian environmental protection.

Probability of Health Effect Given Exposure

This is the central part of health risk assessment, and it entails the NRC paradigm (NRC 1983) components of hazard identification, dose-response analysis, and risk characterization.

Hazard Identification

Hazard identification is distinct from the earlier step of identification of potential threats in that the aim is to assess the weight of evidence as to an agent's toxicity in humans. For some toxicity end points, such as carcinogenicity, formal schemes for weight-of-evidence classification have been proposed, such as those used by the EPA (1996) and the International Agency for Research on Cancer (IARC 1987).

Dose-Response Analysis

Dose-response analysis for exposure to toxic agents describes how the probability of manifesting a toxic end point varies as a function of the magnitude of exposure. Extensive discussion of the methods for this type of analysis, and their pitfalls and interpretations, have occurred over the last two decades and have recently been summarized by Olin et al. (1995). Some issues of particular importance to the assessment of risks to deployed forces bear mentioning, however.

First, what is needed from a dose-response analysis is more than just a definition of exposure levels that can be considered "safe." In environmental or occupational health regulation, the intent is to eliminate unsafe exposures, but in the military setting, it might be especially necessary to consider possible impacts of exposures that are not classifiable as safe. The reason for this is that such exposures might be unavoidable or might be endured intentionally, and to not consider such exposures might engender a more consequential impact on the health of troops or the success of the military mission. Thus, definition of exposure levels that are expected to engender different levels or severities of toxic responses will be one of the ends to which the results of dose-response analysis will be put. This issue is further discussed by Rodricks (1999, abstracted in Appendix A).

Second, for similar reasons, the establishment of "conservative" estimates of dose-response relations, that is, those designed to err on the side of safety when faced with uncertainty about how to project expected human responses from available data, might not be appropriate for certain military uses. When risks cannot be avoided and decisions are made to accept some risks rather than others, or to bear some risk in furtherance of a more fundamental military objective, it is important to make these trade-off decisions with unbiased estimates of the impacts of various courses of action. In other applications, such as the setting of health-protective exposure standards for application in less severe circumstances, conservative estimates might be much more acceptable and indeed desirable. In essence, these are actually questions about the risk-management application of dose-response analysis. The important point here is that such analyses is conducted and its results presented, so that the different uses appropriate for different risk-management settings can be made.

Dose-response analysis for exposure to infectious agents is one that has developed rapidly in recent years. Advances in modeling strategies and the use of data on infection rates after different dose levels in human volunteers have led to descriptions of dose-response patterns for a number of important microbial agents. Currently, these models are better developed for description of infection rates than they are for describing the probabilities of appearance of disease symptoms among those who are infected. The challenge for the risk assessment of deployed forces will be to account for the fact that many microbial risk questions will be about agents that have not been well studied. Indeed, many disease organisms indigenous to various parts of the world have not been properly recognized and described. Attack rates on local inhabitants might be misleading as indicators of effects on American troops encountering the agents for the first time. The issues and challenges of microbial risk assessment in the context of protection of deployed forces is discussed in a paper commissioned by the NRC for this project (Rose 1999, abstracted in Appendix A).

Interactions. Another point to consider is that deployed troops might be exposed under conditions of physical or psychological stress. The effects of stress on the toxicity of agents is not well understood, but there are indications that stress might potentiate effects of other agents. There is the related issue of the effects expected from simultaneous exposure to several agents. In general, the degree to which the toxicities of different agents can be expected to interact is poorly understood and the matter of some controversy. Experimental approaches to this question can be considered, however, and particular attention needs to be paid to those combinations of agents that are identified as in need of scrutiny. The issues around these matters and experimental approaches that have been taken and can be considered are discussed more thoroughly in a paper commissioned by the NRC for this project (Yang 1999, abstracted in Appendix A). These issues are particularly critical for the program of health protection for deployed troops in view of the controversies that have already arisen regarding the potential association of suites of symptoms in veterans of past conflicts with exposures to mixtures of agents that would not be expected to cause such effects individually.

Dose-Time Analysis. Still another critical question is that of duration of exposure and the importance of dose-rate effects. Many (although by no means all) exposures in environmental and occupational health regulation are chronic, low-level exposures that might be experienced at similar levels day after day, and the experimental approaches taken to test agents for toxic effects tend to reflect this in their consistent patterns of daily exposure. In cases of episodic exposure, however, it is not always clear how to apply assessments based on constant-dose rates. This is an ongoing issue in quantitative health risk assessment, but it applies particularly to troop deployment, where the durations of exposure might be indeterminate (depending on the length of deployment) and where transient episodes of high exposure might be encountered. The question is not simply about applying chronic exposure studies to estimation of risks from more acute exposures to troops—the opposite extrapolation is also of concern in cases in which the acute toxicity of agents might be well studied (such as agents in chemical weapons), but the effects of chronic, low-level exposures might not be. A consistent pitfall is the natural tendency to focus on obvious, known hazardous agents and their properties, such that other important effects may be overlooked.

Two basic approaches have been taken to address the question of duration and dose-rate. The more traditional approach is to consider toxicities appearing after dosing on different time scales as separate phenomena, with each time scale requiring testing and analysis of its own. In this approach, acute toxicity, subchronic toxicity, and chronic toxicity are separately characterized by experiments using single doses (or at least a very few doses repeated for at most a few days), doses repeated over several days to weeks, and doses repeated for a substantial portion of lifetime, respectively; separate assessments of dependence of response on dose level are made for each duration category. An application of this approach designed for the case of deployed forces risk assessment is presented by Rodricks (1999, abstracted in Appendix A). The approach also addresses the need mentioned above for determination of doses associated with different levels of adverse impact, not simply those deemed without undue impact. Rodricks proposes a matrix of dose levels that has the duration categories along one dimension and the levels of severity of toxic response along the other. The tabulated doses are those judged to be great enough that effects of the specified severity levels might begin to be expected to occur among people exposed for the various durations. This kind of approach to the problem has the advantage of providing a straightforward, easily interpreted guide to what might be expected as consequences of roughly categorized patterns of exposure. This guide could be particularly useful for rapid decision-making in emergency situations or during deployments, when the information about an exposure is likely to be approximate regarding level and duration. The disadvantages are that the categories are necessarily rough, that intermediate cases are not easily handled, and that exposures that continue over time but are intermittent or vary in intensity are not really addressed, because it is not clear whether their similarities to acute exposures or chronic ones are most relevant.

An alternative approach to duration and dose-response is to attempt to address both the level and duration of exposure in the description of the dose-response relationship in a way that generalizes not only over dose levels but also over time. This is a more ambitious undertaking, and methods are under ongoing development. An analysis of how such an approach could work is presented by Rozman (1999, abstracted in Appendix A). Rozman notes that toxicity of ongoing exposures is a function of the balance between rates of biologic damage and repair. By observing how the rate of encounter with an agent, and the duration of that encounter, interacts with the time scales of the damage and repair processes, it is possible to generalize the description of the dose patterns necessary to generate a toxic response, and also to define conditions under which constant concentration-time products are expected to produce similar responses and those in which they are not. The advantage of this approach is that it makes use of toxicity data from experiments across a range of durations, integrating them into a single toxicological interpretation, and it provides an avenue to consider more complex patterns of variation in exposure level over time. The disadvantage is that many experiments as currently conducted do not provide good information on the role of time. Moreover, in a field situation, the eventual duration of an exposure might not be known when an agent is first encountered, and so duration categories might have to be rough approximations anyway, as in the first approach. Each approach has its advantages, and it is worthwhile pursuing both lines of analysis for application to assessment of risks to deployed forces.

Risk Characterization

Using the information gleaned from the hazard identification and dose-response analysis steps, quantitative estimates of risk can be generated to provide a general understanding of the type and magnitude of an adverse effect that could be caused under particular circumstances or scenarios. Characterization of the uncertainties associated with these estimates is also an important part of this step. In cases where little quantitative data are available for analysis, qualitative characterizations can be made.

Recognition

As discussed earlier, a view of risk scenarios as trees of unfolding events over time helps to organize thinking about the complex chains of circumstances that lead to environmental releases, exposures, and possible adverse reactions. In this regard, the framework becomes a useful tool in noting which outcomes become more likely and which ones less so, thus guiding actions that might be taken to avoid or ameliorate looming risks. To take advantage of these opportunities, it is necessary to recognize any relevant changes in circumstances. Thus, part of the risk-analysis process should seek out opportunities to gather information for updating or altering the probabilities associated with different outcomes of uncertain processes. Practices to gather such key information can then be designed for use in actual deployment. Analysis of the components of complex risk scenarios to determine which are most responsible for overall uncertainty, and the resolution of which issues could most decrease that uncertainty, will contribute to this.

Environmental Consequences

Some agents released into the environment might persist for long periods, even if they do not pose an immediate threat to troops. This could affect deployed troops in the longer run, and it could become an issue if departing troops were seen as having left a contaminated environment behind. An analysis of environmental persistence of any emissions should therefore be part of the risk analysis.

Incorporation into Standards and Risk-Aware Planning

While defining a risk management program is beyond the scope of the present framework, which is aimed at identification and characterization of risks, it is important to provide a context in which the risk assessment results can be brought to bear on practical actions that may be taken to protect the health of deployed forces. The risk management tasks outlined below constitute the use and application of knowledge about threats to health and safety, and it is important to keep these ends in mind when characterizing risks so that the information obtained is appropriate and useful.

The final step of the ongoing strategic baseline preparation phase of the framework is the incorporation of the understanding of risks generated by the previous steps into planning, design of doctrine and standard procedures, and training. Incorporation involves the parts of risk management that can be conducted in the realm of generalized planning and preparation, by forging procedures, capabilities, and standards that will achieve reductions in threats to troops and establish appropriate decision-making practices that can be put to use in the eventuality of actual deployments. It uses the insights into risks posed by various activities and eventualities to plan how to conduct future operations with minimal unnecessary risk and to protect the health and safety of deployed forces to the maximum extent feasible.

Because the focus of the present framework is risk assessment rather than risk management, the treatment of this aspect will be brief, but it is clearly critical if the information developed about potential threats is to become useful in making changes to achieve improved protection of deployed forces.

Incorporation into Design and Doctrine

This large category of activities is meant to cover all of those opportunities to change and improve the military's means and modes of operation during deployment by taking advantage of the insights into risks and their sources identified in the previous steps. It includes the design of equipment, including protective equipment and detectors, means of transportation, logistical support, and weapons to achieve reductions in risks. An important part of this activity is examination of the hazards associated with operation and maintenance of military equipment as well as the use of pesticides and prophylatic agents, hazards that would fall into the category of those associated with deployment per se, discussed earlier. It also includes design of procedures, development of tactics, and reviews of the way that various missions can be carried out, all with the aim of achieving a low-risk environment during deployment, where exposures to hazards are avoided when possible and effectively defended against when necessary.

Also included is the design of practices and procedures for medical surveillance and the development of capabilities for prophylaxis and treatment regarding adverse health effects associated with deployment activities (see IOM 1999 for further discussion). Questions of personnel selection for deployment based on vulnerabilities to risks would also fall under this rubric. The development of detection and exposure measurement techniques and of protective equipment and procedures are also part of this incorporation step (see NRC 1999a,b for further discussion).

During deployment, as exposure probabilities and the likelihood of impacts of hazards change, many decisions will necessarily be based on data immediately available and whatever store of knowledge and analysis has been assembled beforehand. Procedures for gathering and assembling appropriate information and archived analyses, and for using these to make sound decisions, need to be established as a part of preparedness. The Army's 1998 Risk Management Field Manual (FM 100-14) is an example of this kind of preparation.

Development of Standards

The foregoing design activities are aimed at optimizing ways to modify actions and materiel to avoid as much risk as is feasible, and to deal with the risk that cannot be avoided. Another risk-management approach is to define exposure standards that are deemed to achieve some specified degree of protection, and then to screen activities to assure that these standards are met. Although it is unwise to rely on standards alone as a means of controlling risks to military personnel, setting exposure standards is important in establishing a benchmark for protection of health against expected risks. It provides a straightforward means of defining health-protection goals, monitoring activities to assure that those goals are achieved, and allowing for a quick, relatively nontechnical evaluation of the risk potential of situations that have not received detailed analysis. For operational reasons, procedures for determining whether an activity meets exposure standards are desirable because they are relatively easy to formulate and to implement, and they can serve as guides in situations requiring quick decisions based on scarce information by nontechnical decision-makers. The military already uses exposure standards of various kinds a great deal to ensure safety of ongoing operations and to guide decision-making about the special, more-intensive exposures that might occur in emergencies, some deployments, and combat.

Different kinds of standards are appropriate for different settings. Broadly, it is appropriate to allow for different durations of exposure, because a level tolerable for a short time without ill effect might not be so for ongoing exposure. It is also useful to allow for standards that admit some degree of toxic response but protect against incapacitation or irreversible injury for use in guiding actions in emergencies or when important risk trade-off decisions must be made quickly, such as in combat.

By analogy with occupational standards in the civilian arena, military standards for emergencies and cumulative exposures (such as radiation exposure) are useful. The military's operational exposure standards are intended to allow for ongoing exposure of indefinite duration during the conduct of "normal" operations without ill effect, where "normal" means having to do with usual ongoing duties and activities, including military occupational activities. One could imagine a special set of operational exposure standards with assumptions appropriate to limited-term deployments or deployment-specific activities, but in practice the military's usual operational exposure limits fulfill the intent of this kind of standard.

The Short-Term Chemical Exposure Guidelines for Deployed Military Personnel (ACHPPM 1999) are aimed at defining higher exposure levels that can be tolerated in a deployment situation with low likelihood of marked response. They use some military-specific exposure factors but do not make any special consideration for the effect of stress or other deployment-specific factors that might modify sensitivity to agents. They are also aimed at specifying relatively safe levels.

The scheme for reporting risk-assessment results proposed by Rodricks (1999; abstracted in Appendix A) suggests an approach to defining standards that acknowledges that in some situations one must bear adverse effects from exposures to accomplish some other end. This approach is seen most clearly in the Emergency Exposure Guidance Levels (NRC 1986, 1993b, 1998), which estimate air concentrations of substances that might produce reversible effects but do not impair ability to respond to an emergency for a period of an hour. Other standards that provide for different levels of tolerance of some toxic effects for various lengths of exposure could be imagined and could prove useful in particular settings.

A caveat raised before is worth repeating here: standards tend to be set on the most obvious end points, but one must beware of overlooking subtle effects from low-level exposures that might accumulate with repeated episodes of exposure or might manifest themselves long after exposure, even though the exposure causes no detectable immediate harm and might be classified as "safe" with respect to the end point on which short-term limits are based. A recent GAO report was critical of existing DOD procedures and doctrine on this question (GAO 1998).

Contingency Plans

The generalized planning aimed at improving capabilities can be supplemented by contingency plans aimed at specific classes of deployments. These would provide insights into what might be expected in deployments in specific world regions under specific conditions and for specific purposes. They serve as templates, complete with bodies of analysis, ready to be consulted in the eventuality that particular deployments come to be considered, and into which the up-to-date, region-specific information can be plugged. This addresses the problem that complex analyses are difficult to carry out quickly and thoroughly, so the degree to which they can be prepared ahead of time increases preparedness.

Training

The effectiveness of efforts to design procedures and equipment to further the cause of risk prevention depends on the proper and efficient actions of the troops, and training can advance this end. Because a large number of reservists are often deployed, they should be included in such training.

Review

In any complex program in which there are many activities that must interact productively to reach the motivating goals, the military should conduct regular reviews of how well its risk-assessment process is working and how its goals are being fulfilled. It is all too easy to carry out the activities on a list of tasks without ever really bringing the results to bear in the way that motivated the efforts in the first place.

SPECIFIC DEPLOYMENT ACTIVITIES

The second major phase of the framework (Figure 5) addresses the use of these risk-assessment activities in actual, specific deployments. The key activities in this phase are to implement plans made in anticipation of deployment (ongoing strategic baseline preparations), update them with information specific to the deployment situation at hand, note the advent of threatening exposures when they actually occur, and activate the appropriate parts of the response plans accordingly. This phase must also include vigilance for exposures that, despite all the planning, were unanticipated. Finally, it must include collection and archiving of samples for future analysis.

Four subphases of activities associated with specific deployments are (1) deployment-specific planning, (2) activities upon arrival, (3) activities during deployment, and (4) deployment-termination activities.

Deployment-Specific Planning

Once a specific deployment is anticipated, but before it actually occurs, there is an opportunity to apply information specific to the location, mission, and current conditions, and to update and render specific the more generalized contingency plans that might have been developed in the first phase.

The kinds of information that can be applied include current meteorological conditions and forecasts for the immediate future, updates on the locations of hazardous materials, and current assessments of the capabilities and inclinations of any adversaries that might be met. The ongoing strategic baseline analyses divided inventories of threats into those related to deployment per se, those specific to mission types, and those specific to places. The advantage of such a classification is that, when faced with a particular deployment, a situation-specific catalog of hazards can be created by taking all of the first list and adding those from the second and third lists that are appropriate to the particular mission and location. This situation-specific information can then be integrated into the earlier anticipatory analyses as part of the process of mission analysis and planning.

Biological specimens and health-status determinations are helpful tools in monitoring troops' exposures and health, and it is important to establish baseline levels among troops slated for deployment. Baseline information could be obtained by conducting annual health evaluations on reserve and active-duty personnel. Considerations for use of biological markers are discussed in much more detail in a paper commissioned for this project by the NRC (Lippmann 1999, abstracted in Appendix A). Lippmann argues that environmental and biological samples are a good deal less expensive to collect and archive than they are to analyze, and immediate analysis necessarily focuses on agents recognized at the time of collection as being of interest. It is therefore wise to archive most samples and to analyze them only once a specific hypothesis is formed that requires deeper investigation and specific analytical methods.

Activities Upon Arrival

The arrival of the deployed force might provide the first opportunity to collect on-the-ground intelligence. This should include obtaining local samples of soil, air, and water. Some of these should be archived to serve as baseline measures for future reference, but a subset should be analyzed to provide information on the extent and identity of local environmental pollution. Appropriate detection and meteorological instrumentation can be set up to provide the basis for feeding information into exposure models.

Activities During Deployment

This subphase also comprises the main part of the second phase of the risk-assessment framework. During the course of deployment, the key issue is detection of potential exposures and recognition of when situations and contexts occur for which useful prior analysis has been conducted. In the ongoing strategic baseline planning, hypothetical scenarios and schemes for the unfolding of possible threats, the consequences of each threat realized, and the likelihood that hazardous situations would be encountered.

Presumably, plans were formulated for appropriate responses to a range of various eventualities. During an actual deployment, the task is to discern which of the sets of contingent events imagined beforehand are actually transpiring and need a response. This is not merely the detection of agents of concern in the environment, it is the larger question of recognizing the determinants of the changing probabilities that various hazards will be encountered and will pose threats, and modifying actions accordingly.

Detection of Exposures

The detection of imminent exposures is an important aspect of during-deployment activity. (See NRC [1999a] for a discussion of detection methodology and capabilities.) The issue here is how such information can be used. A hierarchy of exposure information could be obtained. First is qualitative detection, which might be provided by a monitoring device that sounds an alarm when a concentration above a certain cutoff is detected. Such detection could trigger actions to employ protective equipment or to take evasive action, but it does not allow such actions to be modulated by the magnitude of the exposure. In many situations, this might not be a significant handicap, because the critical issue is the fact that exposure occurs at all. Next in the hierarchy is the measurement of a concentration (either instantaneously or averaged over some moderate interval). This kind of detection allows different actions depending on whether the concentration is high or low. There is no time component, however, so no allowance for the eventual duration of exposure or the particular concentration-time profile can be made, unless the time course can be guessed from the nature of the source of exposure. A yet more sophisticated detector might be able to keep track of the changing profile of concentration over time. Even if the time-concentration profile is critical to the toxic response engendered, information about the profile becomes complete only after the exposure is completed, and so such information might be of reduced value as a basis for modifying actions to avoid risk. If such profile information is recorded and saved, however, it might be valuable for dosimetry purposes in a retrospective analysis of the impacts of the exposure on the troops who experienced it.

Vigilance for Unsuspected Exposures

Detectors register the presence of those agents they are designed to detect, and prior analyses of threats address the situations that were anticipated, but necessarily exclude possible unexpected exposures. Detecting these in the short run is a challenge, because detection methods would have to be general enough to register whatever agents appear, yet not so general as to react to ubiquitous innocuous compounds. Archived samples might be able to establish previously unsuspected exposures in retrospect. The issues involved in detecting unsuspected exposures, as well as other topics related to preparedness for health protection during deployment, are discussed in a report of the National Science and Technology Council (NSTC 1998).

Sampling, Archiving, and Record Keeping

It is important to take samples over the course of a deployment to document exposures. For practical reasons, the program of sample collection must be tailored to the force size, the nature and duration of the mission, and the type of activities the troops will be called upon to perform. Certain military occupational specialties with known high potential for exposures to particular hazards could be targeted for special attention in personal biological sampling and health surveillance. As noted, it is probably wisest to archive most of these samples until specific questions arise that require their analysis. It should be borne in mind that the surveillance methods have strengths and limitations, and appropriate, validated techniques are not always available. The considerations to be kept in mind when using biological markers are reviewed in a paper commissioned for this project (Lippmann 1999, abstracted in Appendix A). Samples are needed of (1) environmental samples to document initial levels and changes in concentrations over time; (2) information on unit activities and positions over time, so that these can be correlated with mapping of concentrations of agents; and (3) archives of the information gathered by monitors and detectors. Given that all of this information is of value chiefly in retrospect, the motivation to keep records and properly archive materials might be limited. It would appear wise to consider a moderate demand for such activity, but to act to ensure that that modest task is indeed carried out in a context of enormous pressure and demands for successful completion of the military mission. Medical surveillance and record keeping are discussed more fully in a companion report (IOM 1999).

Deployment-Termination Activities

DOD should consider the effectiveness and feasibility of collecting biological samples after deployment for comparison with baseline samples. Challenges in compliance are to be expected, given the troops' personal priorities upon returning home, so sufficiently rigorous enforcement of collection would be needed.

POST-DEPLOYMENT ACTIVITIES

The third and final phase of the overall risk-assessment framework (Figure 6) is the post-deployment phase. This includes the ongoing targeted medical surveillance of deployed veterans to identify late-appearing effects and analyze possible associations of exposure with later health experiences. These activities are discussed in more detail in IOM (1999). The focus here is on the gathering of information that can be fed back to ongoing research on the health and safety risks of deployment.

Enough information must be taken and carefully archived to facilitate reconstruction and tracking of troops' exposures over the course of deployment. The degree to which such exposure reconstruction can occur at the level of individuals or at the level of units depends on the amount of detail available in the records. Among the techniques that can be employed are to assess current exposures to groups that may be similarly exposed or exposed to agents with similar properties, to employ modeling of emissions and environmental fate to reconstruct environmental concentration estimates, and to estimate variation in exposure among individual troops through records of tasks and occupations they experienced during deployment together with estimates of typical exposure while conducting those activities. Exposure assessment approaches are discussed further in a companion report (NRC 1999a).

In a sense, all post-deployment activity is deployment-specific in that it focuses on examining the history and progress of veterans of particular actions. In another sense, however, it is not specific, in that it should be part of a program of following each person through his or her military career and beyond, maintaining job and exposure histories to track all of the factors that are thought likely to be relevant to health protection and the discovery of hazards. Each person will have been involved in a range of activities, and each person's health experience should be examined in the light of that whole history, integrated over specific episodes, including specific deployments. The issues involved with medical surveillance and record-keeping are further discussed in a companion report (IOM 1999).

It seems that possible environmental correlates of disease always bring out alarm-raisers and debunkers, whose public statements can raise public awareness of controversy about the analysis and interpretation of human experience. In view of the objectives of this framework to foster confidence in DOD's reputation as being diligent and responsible in its investigation of the potential causes of health complaints, DOD will have to think carefully about how it will conduct its own surveillance and retrospective analyses and how it will report on these matters to deployed veterans and to the public.

Several particular aspects of post-deployment activities are listed below.

- Immediate attention to the process of reintegrating troops returning from deployment into their normal military life, and reintegrating veterans into the civilian world, might help deal with some of the psychological strains that have proved to be issues in past deployments.
- Systematic processes for the collection and archiving of samples and data should be prepared before they are needed, and put into place promptly to receive data from new deployments. Constructing such mechanisms is really a part of ongoing strategic baseline planning, and setting up systems should not be done in an ad hoc way for each deployment case. It is important to establish a follow-up system, so the appropriate retrospective look at the deployment experience gets carried out systematically.
- Methods should be established to link the ongoing records of the health history of deployed veterans to the deployments that they participated in. Again, this should account for the total history of each person, rather than having records segregated by deployment. The methods should be established permanently rather than set up ad hoc for particular deployments.
- It is important that DOD take advantage of the data on human experiences with the hazards encountered during deployment and conduct ongoing studies. Unit activities data, archived monitoring data, and environmental and biological samples can be used to reconstruct estimates of doses, and these can be examined for association with disease patterns using epidemiological analyses. Hypotheses generated by these studies can then be examined with new tests and toxicological studies, as appropriate.

The points of the above exercises in surveillance and epidemiological analysis are, first, to maintain the ongoing responsibility of the military for the health of its personnel, and second, to learn from past experiences to provide better means for health and safety protection for future deployments. This pursuit can deepen understanding of known threats by adding data from actual experiences. It can in principle help to identify unanticipated threats and call attention to their need for further analysis. All of this information should be fed back to an ongoing process of recognizing and understanding the spectrum of potential threats to the health and safety of deployed U.S. forces. Responsibilities and policy for medical surveillance are given in the 1997 Deployment Medical Surveillance Directive 6490.2. Issues surrounding systematic approaches to post-deployment health surveillance, including the question of how to capture key information to feed back to characterization of incompletely understood health risks, are further discussed in NSTC (1998) and in a companion to the present report (IOM 1999).

SUMMARY AND CONCLUSIONS

Two general approaches could be used to organize a program to improve health protection from hazards that may be encountered in the military environment. One is to organize the risk analysis around hazards. When hazards are recognized, they are characterized and dose-response relationships determined, leading to definition of exposure levels that are deemed acceptable. These acceptable levels are expressed as standards, and activities that might lead to exposures and control measures to limit such exposures can be assessed as to whether they lead to the standards being exceeded, or the costs and effectiveness of various control strategies can be examined and the risks and benefits weighed. This mode of analysis is most appropriate when the nature and magnitude of exposures are well established and predictable, especially when exposures are ongoing.

A second approach is to organize the activities not around the hazards per se, but rather around the activities that one wants to conduct. This second broad approach is most appropriate when the activities can entail a number of different hazards, especially those that might or might not arise depending on the unknown future course of events. The activities are examined to improve understanding about the situations when hazards might manifest themselves and the likelihoods that those situations will arise. The exposures themselves are quite uncertain, and the risks of adverse outcomes are as much a product of the likelihood of the events leading to exposures as they are of the likelihood of adverse responses given that exposure occurs. A typical example of this approach is the fault-tree analysis of potential failures of a nuclear power plant, including a range of modes and amounts of releases that might follow different failure events, and the different environment fates of released materials depending on weather conditions at the unknown time of release. In such an analysis, the risk question is more about the probabilities of exposures of different numbers of people than about the health risk to a person given a certain exposure. Moreover, the whole spectrum of kinds of plant failure needs to be considered together, because adverse outcomes can arise in a number of ways.

Many of the hazards faced in deployment of U.S. forces are of this latter type, with the assessment of risks depending on the analysis of the uncertain events in exposure scenarios and the contingency on the course of events. Moreover, a key objective is to undertake a systematic evaluation of the sources of potential adverse effects, not simply a scanning of activities and scenarios for potential incidents of unacceptably high exposure to known hazards, and the chief challenge in this task is imagining the circumstances, activities, and agents, perhaps in combination, that might lead to health and safety concerns and thus require further investigation and analysis.

The risk-assessment framework proposed in this chapter is a structured approach to gathering, organizing, and analyzing information in a way that encourages a comprehensive, integrated approach to the analysis of threats to deployed troops. As shown in Figures 1 to 6, the framework is characterized by a variety of component parts in which different types of risk-assessment activities are conducted. The organization scheme provides a rational structure for the overall risk-assessment process so that several things become clearer in the whole scheme: where each component activity falls, how each component contributes to the achievement of the ultimate goals, where each analysis takes its input information from, and where its results are used.

In general, the framework can be thought of as a scheme for how DOD can organize a comprehensive and integrated program. The framework is divided into three major categories—ongoing, during deployment, and post-deployment. The ongoing strategic baseline phase covers activities that should be done to prepare for possible future deployments. The first major step is to identify all of the major threats that deployed troops could encounter. The aim is to recognize the array of threats that require further analysis and set them in the context of the activities and settings that prompt them. Several parallel examinations—based on known hazards, notable exposures, and exposures associated with activities and settings directly—should be conducted, and from the combined results of these examinations, an inventory should be created of the agents and exposures and the relative needs for more detailed risk analysis.

After identifying potential hazards to deployed troops, the next step is to develop priorities for which hazards have the greatest likelihood of being encountered and pose the greatest threats to the military mission and to troop health. This task should be based on extant information, experience, and judgment to give the military a rough but rational sequence of hazards to assess.

When priorities have been set, the tools of risk assessment can be applied to quantitatively characterize the hazards, exposures, and outcomes. At this stage, the projected or estimated release, of exposure given release, of health effects given exposure, of certain scenarios unfolding, and of environmental consequences are all used to develop an overall scheme to identify realistic scenarios for given events. The practice of quantitative health risk assessment is best developed for questions concerning exposure to chemical agents and radiation, but can also be applied to microbial threats. For threats from accidents of various descriptions, actuarial data are the best guide, because a large body of documented experience is available and applicable to future settings. The results of these types of analyses can then be incorporated into planning, design of doctrine and standard procedures, and training. The framework does not provide a useful way to estimate combat casualties, which must still be derived from experience, military judgment, and the analysis of war-game results.

The second major phase of activities occurs when a specific deployment is anticipated. At that stage, the generalized contingency plans developed on an ongoing basis can be refined and made more specific, based on the known location, the type of mission, and current conditions. Once deployment occurs, health and environmental data should be collected, monitored, and archived, if feasible. The data could be used for real-time risk decisions and later reconstruction of exposure scenarios. An important aspect of this step is the identification of exposures and outcomes that were not previously anticipated.

Post-deployment risk-assessment activities comprise the third major phase of the framework. In this phase, when troops and reserves are reintegrated back into their garrison or civilian lives, it is important to continue surveillance of veterans' health and to study any uncertain outcomes using exposure reconstruction and epidemiological analyses. Much of the information obtained during this phase can then be used to refine earlier risk analyses and to search for or study threats not previously considered.

It is presumed that the various component analyses of the framework will be executed in good faith and interpreted carefully, with full awareness of the possibilities and shortcomings of the available methods. The framework concentrates on how the results of all of these activities can come together, how they can be pursued systematically to ensure that important aspects are not overlooked, and how they become useful in addressing the overall objectives of the larger enterprise.

Although the degree to which current DOD activities and programs fulfill the approaches recommended here will be important in implementation of this framework, implementation would not be a simple exercise in checking off components on a list. What makes the framework relevant is not the execution of each of its elements, however competently done, but rather the systematic approach to the process of assessing threats to deployed troops and incorporating the results of each element of analysis into an integrated program that addresses the overall objectives of the troop health-protection program. Only by keeping these ends in mind and continually evaluating the collective effectiveness of the risk-analysis activities in meeting them will the individual component activities play their needed role in the overall program.

5

Considerations and Recommendations for Implementing the Framework

AREAS OF EMPHASIS FOR IMPLEMENTING THE FRAMEWORK

Given the scope of this undertaking, which demands a risk-assessment framework covering a diverse array of sources of threats to the health and safety of deployed U.S. forces, the approach presented in this report is necessarily broad and expressed in general terms. What has been proposed is truly a framework rather than a set of procedures or methods for actually conducting the analyses; that is, it is a structured context for organizing risk-assessment activities, ensuring their completeness, and aligning them with the motivating needs and questions.

The Department of Defense (DOD) has an extensive set of organizational units implementing a variety of sophisticated programs in which data are collected, capabilities are developed, and analyses are conducted and applied to the protection of troops. However, as mentioned in Chapter 1, it is beyond the scope of this study to review all of the current activities that comprise DOD's structure and activities for protecting the health of deployed forces. Such a review of existing practices would be valuable, however, and it should focus not only on the array of capabilities, but on an assessment of how effectively these capabilities and existing activities come together to form a comprehensive program. Even before such a review, some areas can be identified that need greater DOD emphasis.

In general, there is a natural tendency to focus attention on hazardous agents already known. Although it is important to characterize known hazards, too much emphasis on this aspect may result in overlooking other hazards that, with some attention, could have been recognized. A good part of the motivation for examining DOD's risk efforts is to establish how to avoid surprises about the toxicity of deployment exposures and to address questions that might arise even after diligent and responsible attempts have been made to ensure the protection of troops' health. Therefore, it is important that the framework include a systematic approach to discover unrecognized potential hazards and to highlight areas with inadequate information to determine whether a potential for risk exists. Among the many exposures and activities associated with deployment, it is likely that relatively few will pose previously unrecognized threats to health and safety, but it is just as important to establish the lack of a hazard for the many cases as it is to recognize the potential hazards of the few that do entail notable risks.

A similar pitfall is to attend to the known or principal toxic effects of an agent while failing to give proper attention to delayed, less-pronounced or less-frequent adverse consequences, or previously unrecognized effects—especially those that might arise from patterns of exposure other than those that called attention to the agent in the first place. For example, a great deal of attention has been focused on the acute toxicity of chemical warfare agents and the amounts and patterns of exposure that would lead to immediate battlefield casualties if troops were to be attacked with such agents. However, rather little attention seems to have been given to the potential for delayed chronic toxicity, either as a consequence of surviving such an attack or from exposures to much lower levels of the agents, as might be experienced by many troops outside the zone where concentrations are sufficient to be of immediate military concern.

Another aspect of particular concern in deployments, and one that has arisen in questions about health consequences of past deployments, is that of co-exposure to two or more agents simultaneously, including questions about exposures under conditions of physical and psychological stress. Past experience with hazardous agents, toxicity testing, and conventional risk analysis have all focused on assessing exposures one at a time, and this course of analysis might leave one unprepared to recognize the potential hazards generated when substantial exposures to several agents are experienced together.

A final special aspect of risk analysis for deployment is the large role that risk-risk comparisons must play. Given the high level of tactical risk that might be inherent in the deployment situation, some health and safety risks may be appropriate to avoid or mitigate even greater risks. Determining how to optimize the trade-offs requires simultaneous consideration of the spectrum of risks faced by deployed troops, along with the possibility that actions taken to avoid or ameliorate some risks might exacerbate others.

All of those factors suggest that an agent-by-agent approach—focusing on determining acceptable exposure levels to each recognized hazard—might not, by itself, be sufficient for the need to assess risks to deployed forces. The framework proposed in this report has attempted to address this issue by devoting considerable attention to analyses of the activities, materials uses, and settings of deployment, and to the recognition of the situations under which potentially hazardous exposures might arise.

The agent-by-agent approach is used to organize much of the risk analysis conducted to support environmental regulation. When hazards are recognized, they are characterized and dose-response relationships are determined. Exposure levels that are deemed acceptable are then defined. These acceptable levels are expressed as standards, and activities that might lead to exposures and control measures to limit such exposures can be assessed in relation to the standards. Also, costs and effectiveness of various control strategies can be examined and the risks and benefits weighed. This mode of analysis is most appropriate when the nature and magnitude of exposures are well established and predictable, especially when exposures are ongoing.

An alternative approach, which is the focus of the proposed framework, is to organize efforts not around the hazards per se but rather around the probable activities of deployed troops. Such an approach is most appropriate when the activities can entail a number of different hazards, especially those that might arise from the unknown course of future events. The activities are examined to understand situations when hazards might manifest themselves and the likelihoods that those situations will arise. This is because the exposures themselves are quite uncertain, and the risks of adverse outcomes are as much a product of the likelihood of events leading to exposure as of the likelihood of adverse responses given that such exposures occur.

A typical example of this approach is the fault-tree analysis of potential failures of a nuclear power plant. A fault-tree analysis includes alternative modes and amounts of releases that might occur depending on different failure events, and the different fates of released material in the environment depending on weather conditions at the unknown time of release. In such an analysis, the risk question is more about the probabilities of exposures of different numbers of people than about the health risk to a person given a certain exposure. Moreover, the whole spectrum of kinds of plant failure needs to be considered together, because adverse outcomes can arise in a number of ways.

Many of the hazards faced in deployment are best represented by this latter approach, with the assessment of risks depending as much on the analysis of uncertain events. Moreover, a key objective is to undertake a systematic evaluation of the sources of potential adverse effects, not simply a scanning of activities and scenarios for potential incidents of unacceptably high exposure to known hazards. The chief challenge in this task is imagining the circumstances, activities, and agents—perhaps in combination—that might lead to health and safety concerns, and thus require further investigation and analysis.

These considerations suggest that a framework organized largely around analyses of activities and settings might be appropriate for the present purposes. A good deal of emphasis is placed on recognition of potentially risk-generating situations and on constructing sets of scenarios under which adverse effects could manifest themselves. Nonetheless, analysis of these scenarios requires that they be decomposed into elements that are amenable to investigation by established exposure assessment and health risk analysis tools. The four-step NRC (1983) paradigm remains at the heart of the framework, albeit expanded somewhat to consider the role of uncertainties and contingencies in the events leading to exposures.

A large armamentarium of analytical techniques appropriate to the various constituent tasks of risk analysis has been developed through extensive practice and ongoing debate among practitioners and the larger affected community over the last decades. Although the application and interpretation of these techniques for the military's purposes—and in particular for the assessment of threats to deployed forces—need to be carefully considered, this examination is best done in the context of the larger framework. The aims of the framework are to try to ensure that the methods and analyses follow from DOD's ultimate objectives and to clarify how the results obtained bear on achieving those objectives.

MEETING THE STATED OBJECTIVES FOR THE FRAMEWORK

A set of objectives for a risk-assessment framework for deployed U.S. forces was proposed in Chapter 2. The following items discuss the benefits that could be realized by implementing the framework to meet those objectives.

- By focusing on the analysis of the hazards associated with particular deployment activities, the framework aims at enhancing the efficiency with which potential threats can be identified and characterized. Moreover, it acts to tie the analysis of threats directly to the activities and settings where they may operate, and organizing the analysis to facilitate integrated study of the spectrum of hazards that need to be considered in developing improved practices and equipment. This enables and encourages the development of plans and designs that minimize overall impact, rather than ad hoc adjustments to existing processes to ensure that this or that exposure standard is not violated. This structure encourages true optimization and efforts at continuous improvement.

- The framework proposed in this report is designed to provide a structure that ensures systematic progression through all of the tasks and requirements of the many programs and activities that DOD already has in place. It is also aimed at showing how all of the pieces fit together to contribute to the overall goals. It provides a context for evaluating the effectiveness of efforts to address the needs of the overall program.
- The framework encourages assiduous search for potential hazards and recognition of situations in which risks to health and safety might arise. There is a large emphasis on investigation, planning, and design carried out prospectively, not just in reaction to problems that might arise. By having an organized, vigorous program to identify and characterize threats, DOD can establish its interest in prevention and forthrightly address risk issues.
- The organizing principle of the framework encourages awareness of the potential risks in all activities by examining the consequences of those activities. Thus, risk considerations are not simply added on as extra requirements or constraints on design of procedures and materiel, they are an integral part of such design. The framework calls on analysts to think through all activities to identify conditions that might lead to encountering hazards, which can lead to recognition of potential but not immediately obvious risks.
- By making protection from hazards an integral part of planning and training, the readiness and capabilities produced are known to military personnel. The existence of a comprehensive program can foster confidence among the troops that their health and safety are taken seriously and that the risks they are asked to bear are minimized and justified.
- The framework provides for sample-taking and record keeping that will permit post hoc reconstruction of deployment exposures should the need arise for analysis of potential links of exposures with health outcomes. It calls for systematic procedures to gain from the experience of deployments as they occur. By emphasizing prior planning and recognizing previously uncharacterized hazards, the framework aims at minimizing the chances that consequential risk factors are overlooked, and it provides evidence that a systematic, thorough, good-faith effort is continually made to identify, characterize, and avoid sources of threats to the health and safety of deployed forces.

- The need to balance measures taken to protect against hazards with military concerns and with the other risks that these measures might engender is considered throughout the framework. By explicitly considering hazards in the context of the activities and settings in which they arise, and by considering all of the various hazardous aspects of an activity in one analysis, this framework encourages making the kind of risk-risk comparisons and optimization of design of procedures that are required to achieve protection without undue burdens. By characterizing the impacts of various levels of exposure, and not simply defining safe levels, the ability to make appropriate trade-offs is enhanced. The framework attempts to structure the risk-assessment activities to enhance the utility of the results for the risk-management process.

Implementing a framework such as that proposed in the present report is a significant challenge. It is intended that the framework provide a structure and context for organizing current DOD risk assessment activities, and is not necessarily a suggestion for developing new activities. The challenge of implementation will be to ensure that as an operating plan is developed, the conceptual organization and ties among activities that the framework attempts to foster are captured in the practical organization of the workforce, its tasks, and its missions. DeRoos et al. (1988) have provided a useful set of observations on organizing a work force for assessing environmental health risks. This includes listing the necessary skills, training, and specialization of workers, and stresses that accomplishing the larger ends is a function of the appropriate interaction of (1) the skills of personnel, (2) the definition and organization of the tasks they carry out, including appropriate interaction and teamwork among personnel, and (3) the work organization objectives. The present framework attempts to address the third aspect of developing a strategy for assessing risks in the context of the constraints and challenges of deployment. To reiterate a point made earlier in the present report, what makes the framework relevant is not the execution of each of its elements, however competently done. Only by keeping the ends and goals in mind and continually evaluating the collective effectiveness of the risk-analysis activities in meeting them will the individual component activities play their needed role in the overall program.

Risk assessment should never be a process of blindly following the results of prescribed analyses; sound analysis will always require the exercise of considerable professional and expert judgment. Risk assessment is a tool in exercising such judgment, not a replacement for it. The importance of judgment, and the need to apply it in an open and frank manner, if risk analyses are to gain wide support and public confidence, are stressed in several recent panel reports (NRC 1994, 1996; PCCRARM 1997a,b). The recommendations below should be viewed in this light.

RECOMMENDATIONS

1. A Risk-Assessment Framework

DOD should consider the risk-assessment framework presented in this report as a basis for organizing its efforts to protect the safety and health of forces deployed in hostile environments.

The proposed framework presented in Chapter 4 constitutes the major recommendation of this report. The recommendations that follow apply to the further development and implementation of the framework.

2. Objectives for the Framework

DOD should develop an explicit list of objectives, such as illustrated in this report, for its efforts to protect the health and safety of deployed forces.

Because a risk-assessment framework for action should be designed to achieve objectives, a fully realized framework cannot be constructed until those objectives are clearly articulated. Although lofty goals are admirable and might be useful in defining a vision, simply stating a set of ideals to be striven for is not, by itself, sufficient. It is important that the objectives deal with the practical difficulties that will be encountered and set out how the conflicts among objectives will be dealt with.

The objectives should serve as part of a strategic plan for DOD to increase trust among the public and among military personnel that matters of health and safety from deployment activities are being forthrightly and competently addressed. The plan should be followed by specific, active measures.

Also, the objectives should be practical, concrete, and measurable. Measurement of progress would serve as an index to the adequacy of the framework and efforts to implement it.

3. DOD's Special Responsibilities

DOD should examine and analyze the military's special responsibilities for protection of its personnel and how these responsibilities differ from those of a typical employer, manufacturer, or regulator.

The aim here is to define what DOD's duty is regarding protection of its personnel and what it might be held accountable for in retrospect.

These matters are as much moral, social, and philosophical as they are technical, and the question should be approached accordingly. The risk-assessment framework should then be refined to reflect those special responsibilities.

Issues to be considered include the unusual degree of control the military has over the actions and exposures of its personnel; the need to call for individual troops to put life, limb, and health at risk in the interests of the military mission and the nation at large; the problems of trading off possibilities of health effects in later life with immediate risks of casualties and impacts on military mission or military capabilities; and other matters in which the equity and voluntariness of risk-bearing arise.

If the risk analysis is to effectively contribute to such decisions, it will require an articulation of a doctrine on how risk trade-offs are to be considered. In addition, DOD should attempt to articulate a set of principles on how the balance of long-term risks to the troops and risks to the military mission should be approached. This effort should also address the nature of responsibilities for the post-deployment and post-career health of personnel, and appropriate standards for treatment or compensation of personnel who are possibly affected by exposures to hazards suffered during deployment.

4. The Capacity to Recognize New Hazards

DOD's efforts to assess risks from deployment activities should include a substantial effort to recognize previously unappreciated hazards and to examine the activities and potential settings for deployment to determine where hazards might arise.

Although more fully characterizing known hazards and the circumstances under which they arise is essential to effective mitigation of risks, these efforts should not blind the program to the possibilities of novel hazards. Attention to this task is essential for providing for measures to reduce the chances that exposures come into question after the fact, as well as for meeting those cases that might nonetheless arise with evidence that appropriate diligence in evaluating safety issues was exercised. Activities and settings of potential deployment should be pursued by systematically examining the contexts in which exposures that need investigation might arise.

5. A Full Consideration of the Toxic Effects of Harmful Agents

DOD should attend to all of the effects of a hazardous agent, not only the principal ones or those that called attention to the agent as a hazard in the first place.

In particular, attention should be paid to the possibility that long-term or delayed chronic effects might result from exposures to agents that are examined mainly for their acute toxicity. Frequently, the possibility of such latent effects has been poorly examined, but the lack of data should not be confused with a presumption that no effects exist. The natural tendency to regard acutely toxic agents only as potential sources of immediate casualties should be tempered by this realization. Another important consideration is low-level exposure as a possible cause of chronic toxicity.

6. Extrapolating Information on Toxic Effects

DOD should continue to conduct research and develop methods to improve its capabilities to extrapolate information on toxic effects to address the full variety of magnitudes, durations, patterns, and co-exposures that might be encountered during deployment.

The problems of extrapolating toxic effects across different patterns of concentration and time are particularly important to the assessments the military must carry out. Exposures can range from a single event to chronic exposures over long periods. Similarly, possible effects can become apparent over different times, including rapid response and long-delayed response.

7. Psychological and Physical Stress

Risk-assessment methods need to be developed to characterize and predict effects of stress, so that this dimension can be integrated into the analysis of the spectrum of threats faced by deployed forces.

The roles of psychological and physical stress in potentiating or exacerbating the toxicity of physical, chemical, and biological agents and as hazards in their own right are not well understood, but their role in the deployment situation is potentially large. DOD has an opportunity and a need to become a leader in the study of stress and its interaction with toxicity. Moreover, stress itself as a sufficient cause of adverse health effects is relatively poorly understood despite substantial and convincing evidence that it is common among deployed troops.

8. Microbial Agents

DOD should conduct research and develop methods to assess risks from exposure to microbial agents and should strive to characterize the variety of disease organisms—and troops' vulnerabilities to them—that might be encountered around the world.

Despite recent major advances, the ability to assess quantitative risks of adverse health outcomes from exposure to microbial agents is in need of further research and development of methodology, an area in which DOD could play a large role that would also be of service to the larger risk-assessment community. This would permit the incorporation of microbial threats into risk-risk tradeoff comparisons.

9. Anticipating Potentially Harmful Exposures

Intentional or unintentional exposures that result from the procedures, equipment, and activities associated with maintaining a presence in an unusual environment should be scrutinized for potential threats to the health of deployed troops.

Many and perhaps most of the hazards encountered during deployment are ascribable to the activities, agents, and materials of deployment per se or to the risks inherent in the tasks of the military mission. DOD should continue its efforts to document hazards associated with places around the globe as a contingency for possible future deployments. This should include documentation of the use and storage of toxic industrial chemicals, identification and characterization of indigenous infectious diseases, and descriptions of local environmental pollution and contamination. It should also include assessments of hazards posed by terrain and infrastructure and the accumulation of climate, meteorological, and hydrological data for use in fate and transport modeling of potential releases.

10. Exposures to Mixtures

DOD should undertake special examination of patterns of co-exposure.

Deployment might entail simultaneous exposures to a number of hazards, and possible toxicological synergism among agents has played an important role in debates about health effects among veterans of past deployments. This is a rising issue in the arena of risk assessment generally, raised by mandates of the 1996 Food Quality Protection Act. DOD has an opportunity and a need to be a leader in developing approaches to this question, including practical means to identify important co-exposures, methods for assessing cumulative risk, and approaches to testing for health effects resulting from co-exposures. Consideration should be given to the role of prophylactic substances that might be part of the combined exposures.

11. Exposure Scenario Development

In cases of hazardous agents for which the possibility and degree of exposure to troops is uncertain due to dependence on circumstances and events that vary widely from case-to-case, DOD should create scenarios describing the possible chain of events leading to exposure to troops.

For many hazards of interest in the assessment of risks to deployed forces, the key question for analysis is not about the health effects of a certain exposure, but about the likelihood that the events will produce that exposure. DOD should consider approaching such questions by creating scenarios describing the possible chains of events leading to exposures of troops, and then quantitatively assessing the likelihood of alternative courses of events, as further described in Chapter 4. There may be some advantage in using a standard set of scenarios for broad classes of hazards, with additional details as needed for specific hazards.

12. Biological Markers

DOD should conduct research on developing appropriate biological markers of exposure and effect for surveillance of those exposures that are of particular relevance to the deployment setting.

13. Identifying Different Degrees of Exposure and Impact

As an aid to quick decision-making when emergencies arise from particular hazardous exposures, DOD should identify a series of exposure levels and durations at which individuals are expected to begin to suffer progressively severe effects.

To be useful for assessing settings in which some levels of risk must be borne, it is necessary that quantitative risk analysis not confine itself to identification of safe or acceptable levels of exposure alone; it is also necessary to characterize the different degrees of impact that one might expect at levels of exposure that exceed levels that would normally be thought of as safe. A simple scheme such as that suggested by Rodricks (1999) should be considered, in which exposure levels are identified that begin to produce adverse effects of different levels of severity in some individuals among an exposed group. This approach captures the main features of the quantitative relationship and provides a quick guide that is useful in making time-critical judgments regarding risk trade-offs, an important ability in the deployment context. For such guides to be effective in practice, a clear layout of decision-making responsibility and authority is necessary.

14. A Risk-Management Framework

DOD should consider developing an explicit framework for risk-management decision-making.

A risk-management framework would bring the risks characterized by the risk-assessment framework proposed in this report to bear on the improvement of procedures, doctrine, and materiel to diminish unnecessary risk as far as possible; to reduce risks that cannot be avoided; and to make rational, informed decisions about how to optimize action in the face of risks and uncertainties that cannot be eliminated. The tools of operations research and decision analysis are applicable, including value of information analysis, benefit-cost analysis, cost-effectiveness analysis, and multiattribute utility theory.

15. Determining Whether DOD's Objectives Are Met

In considering the present proposed framework for assessing risks to the health and safety of deployed forces, DOD should review its existing activities in this area and determine the degree to which they fulfill its objectives.

It is important, however, to go beyond an accounting of the component activities; it is necessary to assess the way in which the various activities come together to address all aspects of protecting the health and safety of deployed forces and to determine how the objectives are being addressed. As stated at the outset, the technical procedures are merely the means to an end. The technical results must be thoughtfully and vigorously applied to the achievement of the articulated objectives.

References

ACHPPM (U.S. Army Center for Health Promotion and Preventive Medicine). 1999. Short-Term Chemical Exposure Guidelines for Deployed Military Personnel. TG230A. Draft. Aberdeen Proving Ground, Edgewood, MD. (March).

Barnthouse, L., J. Fava, K. Humphreys, R. Hunt, L. Laibson, S. Noesen, J. Owens, J. Todd, B. Vigon, K. Weitz, and J. Young. 1997. Life-Cycle Impact Assessment: The State of the Art, 2nd Ed. Pensacola, FL.: Society of Environmental Toxicology and Chemistry (SETAC).

Clemen, R. 1990. Making Hard Decisions. New York, NY: PWT, Kent.

Curran, M.A. 1996. Environmental Life Cycle Assessment. New York: McGraw Hill.

DeRoos R.L., P.N. Anderson, N.J. Berberich, B. Maugans, G.S. Omenn, P.G. Rentos. 1988. Observations on work force and training needs for assessing environmental health risks. Public Health Rep. 103(4):348-354.

DODD (Department of Defense Directive). 1997. Joint Medical Surveillance. Directive 6490.2. Department of Defense. (August 30, 1997.)

Environmental Defense Fund. 1997. Toxic Ignorance: The Continuing Absence of Basic Health Testing for Top-Selling Chemicals in the United States. New York: Environmental Defense Fund.

EPA (United States Environmental Protection Agency). 1987. The Risk Assessment Guidelines of 1986. EPA/600/8-87/045. Washington, D.C.: Office of Health and Environmental Assessment.

EPA (United States Environmental Protection Agency). 1996. Proposed Guidelines for Carcinogen Risk Assessment. EPA/600/P-92/003C. http://www.epa.gov/ORD/WebPubs/carcinogen.

GAO (United States General Accounting Office). 1998. Chemical Weapons: DOD Does Not Have a Strategy to Address Low-Level Exposures. GAO/NSIAD-98-228. Washington, D.C.: United States General Accounting Office.

IARC (International Agency for Research on Cancer). 1987. Pp. 17-34. In: Monographs on the Evaluation of the Carcinogenic Risk of Chemicals to Humans. Overall Evaluations of Carcinogenicity:An Updating of IARC Monographs Volumes 1-42., Supplement 7. Lyon, France: IARC.

IOM (Institute of Medicine). 1999. Strategies to Protect the Health of Deployed U.S. Forces: Medical Surveillance, Record Keeping, and Risk Reduction. Washington, D.C.: National Academy Press.

JSC (Joint Chiefs of Staff). 1998. Memorandum: Deployment Health Surveillance and Readiness. MCM-251-98. Office of the Chairman, Washington, D.C. Dated 4 December 1998.

Kaplan, S. and B.J. Garrick. 1981. On the quantitative definition of risk. Risk Analysis 1(1):11-27.

Lippmann, M. 1999. Approaches for the Collection and Use of Personal-Exposure and Human Biological-Marker Information for Assessing Risks to Deployed U.S. Forces in Hostile Environments. In: Strategies to Protect the Health of Deployed U.S. Forces Workshop Proceedings: Assessing Health Risks to Deployed U.S. Forces. January 28-29, 1999. Washington, D.C.: National Academy Press.

Martin, E. 1999. Characteristics of the Future Battlefield and Deployment. In: Strategies to Protect the Health of Deployed U.S. Forces Workshop Proceedings: Assessing Health Risks to Deployed U.S. Forces. January 28-29, 1999. Washington, D.C.: National Academy Press.

Morgan, M.G. and M. Henrion 1990. Uncertainty : A Guide to Dealing with Uncertainty in Quantitative Risk and Policy Analysis. Cambridge, New York: Cambridge University Press.

NAE (National Academy of Engineering). 1998. The Ecology of Industry: Sectors and Linkages. Washington, D.C.: National Academy Press.

NCEH (National Center for Environmental Health). 1996. Environmental Public Health Surveillance Workshops. Online. Available: http://www.cdc.gov/nceh/programs/ephs/wkshop.

NRC (National Research Council). 1972. The Effects on Populations of Exposure to Low Levels of Ionizing Radiation. Washington, D.C.: National Academy of Sciences.

NRC (National Research Council). 1974. The Effects on Populations of Exposure to Low Levels of Ionizing Radiation. Washington, D.C.: National Academy of Sciences.

NRC (National Research Council). 1980. The Effects on Populations of Exposure to Low Levels of Ionizing Radiation:1980. Washington, D.C.: National Academy Press.

NRC (National Research Council). 1983. Risk Assessment in the Federal Government: Managing the Process. Washington, D.C.: National Academy Press.

NRC (National Research Council). 1986. Criteria and Methods for Preparing Emergency Exposure Guidance Level (EEGL), Short-Term Public Emergency Guidance Level (SPEGL), and Continuous Guidance Level (CEGL) Documents. Washington, D.C.: National Academy Press.

NRC (National Research Council). 1988. Health Risks of Radon and Other Internally Deposited Alpha-Emitters: BEIR IV. Washington, D.C.: National Academy Press.

NRC (National Research Council). 1990. Health Effects of Exposure to Low Levels of Ionizing Radiation: BEIR V. Washington, D.C.: National Academy Press.

NRC (National Research Council). 1993a. Issues in Risk Assessment. Washington, D.C.: National Academy Press.

NRC (National Research Council). 1993b. Guidelines for Developing Community Emergency Exposure Levels for Hazardous Substances. Washington, D.C.: National Academy Press.

NRC (National Research Council). 1994. Science and Judgment in Risk Assessment. Washington, D.C.: National Academy Press.

NRC (National Research Council). 1996. Understanding Risk: Informing Decisions in a Democratic Society. Washington, D.C.: National Academy Press.

NRC (National Research Council). 1998. Standing Operating Procedures of the National Advisory Committee on Acute Exposure Guideline Levels for Hazardous Substances (Draft). Washington, D.C.: National Academy Press.

NRC (National Research Council). 1999a. Strategies to Protect the Health of Deployed U.S. Forces: Technology and Methods for Detection and Tracking of Exposures to a Subset of Harmful Agents. Washington, D.C.: National Academy Press.

NRC (National Research Council). 1999b. Strategies to Protect the Health of Deployed U.S. Forces: Physical Protection and Decontamination. Washington, D.C.: National Academy Press.

NRC (National Research Council). 1999c. Strategies to Protect the Health of Deployed U.S. Forces Workshop Proceedings: Assessing Health Risks to Deployed U.S. Forces. January 28-29, 1999. Washington, D.C.: National Academy Press.

NRC (National Research Council). 1999d. Health Effects of Exposure to Radon: BEIR VI. Washington, D.C.: National Academy Press.

NSTC (National Science and Technology Council). 1998. A National Obligation Planning for Health Preparedness for and Readjustment of the Military, Veterans, and Their Families after Future Deployments. Presidential Review Directive 5 Executive Office of the President, Office of Science and Technology Policy, Washington D.C.

Olin, S., W. Farland, C. Park, L. Rhomberg, R. Scheuplein, T. Starr, and J. Wilson, eds. 1995. Low-Dose Extrapolation of Cancer Risks: Issues and Perspectives. Washington, D.C.: ILSI Press.

PCCRARM (Presidential/Congressional Commission on Risk Assessment and Risk Management). 1997a. Framework for Environmental Health Risk Management. Washington, D.C.

PCCRARM (Presidential/Congressional Commission on Risk Assessment and Risk Management). 1997b. Risk Management in Regulatory Decision-Making. Washington, D.C.

Pojasek, R.B. 1998. P2 assessments: What are they good for? Pollution Prevention Review, 8(4):101-109.

Rhomberg, L.R. 1995. "What Constitutes 'Dose'? (Definitions)" Pp. 185-198, in: Low-Dose Extrapolation of Cancer Risks: Issues and Perspectives. S. Olin, W. Farland, C. Park, L. Rhomberg, R. Scheuplein, T. Starr, and J. Wilson, eds. Washington, D.C.: ILSI Press.

Rhomberg, L.R. 1997. A survey of methods for chemical health risk assessment among federal regulatory agencies. Human and Ecological Risk Assessment, 3(6):1029-1196.

Rodricks, J. 1999. The Nature of Risk Assessment and Its Application to Deployed U.S. Forces. In: Strategies to Protect the Health of Deployed U.S. Forces Workshop Proceedings: Assessing Health Risks to Deployed U.S. Forces. January 28-29, 1999. Washington, D.C.: National Academy Press.

Rose, J. 1999. Future Health Assessment and Risk Management Integration for Infectious Diseases and Biological Agents for Deployed Forces. In: Strategies to Protect the Health of Deployed U.S. Forces Workshop Proceedings: Assessing Health Risks to Deployed U.S. Forces. January 28-29, 1999. Washington, D.C.: National Academy Press.

Rozman, K. 1999. Approaches for Using Toxicokinetic Information in Assessing Risks to Deployed U.S. Forces. In: Strategies to Protect the Health of Deployed U.S. Forces Workshop Proceedings: Assessing Health Risks to Deployed U.S. Forces. January 28-29, 1999. Washington, D.C.: National Academy Press.

Thacker, S.B., D.F. Stroup, R.G. Parrish and H.A. Anderson. 1996. Surveillance in environmental public health: issues, systems, and sources. Am J Public Health. 86(5):633-8.

U.S. Army. 1998. Risk Management. Field Manual FM-100-14. Dept. of the Army, Washington, D.C. (April 23, 1998).

von Winterfeldt, D. and W. Edwards. 1986. Decision Analysis and Behavioral Research. Cambridge, New York: Cambridge University Press.

Weeks, J.L. 1991. Occupational health and safety regulation in the coal mining industry: public health at the workplace. Annu Rev Public Health 12:195-207.

Yang, R. 1999. Health Risks and Preventive Research Strategy for Deployed U.S. Forces from Toxicologic Interactions Among Potentially Harmful Agents. In: Strategies to Protect the Health of Deployed U.S. Forces Workshop Proceedings: Assessing Health Risks to Deployed U.S. Forces. January 28-29, 1999. Washington, D.C.: National Academy Press.

Appendixes

A

Abstracts of Commissioned Papers

Approaches for the Collection and Use of Personal Exposure and Human Biological-Marker Information for Assessing Risks to Deployed U.S. Forces

Morton Lippmann, Ph.D.
New York University School of Medicine, Tuxedo, NY

Abstract

Risk management is especially important for military forces deployed in hostile or chemically contaminated environments. On-line communications or rapid turnaround capabilities for assessing exposures can create viable options for preventing or minimizing incapacitating exposures or latent disease or disability in the years after the deployment. With military support for the development, testing, and validation of state-of-the-art personal and area sensors, telecommunications, and data management resources, the Department of Defense can (1) enhance its capabilities for meeting its novel and challenging tasks and (2) create technologies that will find widespread civilian uses.

This paper assesses currently available options and technologies for productive pre-deployment environmental surveillance, exposure surveillance during deployments, and retrospective post-deployment exposure surveillance. It introduces some opportunities for technological and operational advancements in technology for more effective exposure surveillance and effects management options for force deployments in future years. The issues discussed include: (1) information needs for assessing personal exposures and risks for deployed forces; (2) options for pre-deployment baseline determinations, for collection of personal exposure-related data during field deployment, and for post-deployment personal exposure assessments; (3) maximizing effective personal exposure data resources during deployment and post-deployment; (4) technical capabilities for personal exposure assessment; and (5) assessing risks.

Advances in information technology have made it possible to envision the collection, maintenance, and utilization of deployment data that would enable theater commanders and medical staff to recognize and evaluate environmental health hazards and to manage deployments to avoid or minimize those hazards. Such data, together with a deployment sample archive, would also facilitate future epidemiological studies that could identify additional causal relationships between environmental factors and health outcomes.

Applications can include: (1) on-line communications access to remote sensing devices and continuous monitoring of data for tactical planning; (2) data review by medical staff personnel to determine the need for monitoring military personnel for possible effects of toxic exposures, provide countermeasures during deployments, and set priorities for medical examinations and biomarker sample collections and analyses in the early post-deployment period; (3) additional sampling or monitoring, or analysis of archived samples, to resolve ambiguities or conflicts concerning levels of exposure or environmental contamination; and (4) post-deployment review of medical and environmental data by epidemiologists in investigations of possible causal factors for delayed illness reports associated with service in a specific deployment.

Each of these applications could consume large amounts of resources, and the allocations should be decided according to pre-established priorities by an appropriate panel of peers, including military users and state-of-the-art research investigators with expertise in the emerging technologies.

Characteristics of the Future Battlefield and Deployment

Edward D. Martin, M.D.
Edward Martin and Associates, Inc., Arlington, VA

Abstract

In an era of unprecedented change, the military planner of today must prepare for contingencies involving operations by forces of a very large size to forces for special operations and operations other than war that might involve just a few soldiers, sailors, or airmen. The entire spectrum of geographical features and weather conditions must be accounted for in the plan. The typical linear battlefield will be replaced by a combat situation with a 360-degree threat, the potential for new high-technology weapons, the use of chemical and biological agents, and the use of nontraditional forces and terrorism.

With the gradual urbanization of the world's population, future battles will inevitably be fought within city limits geometrically compounding the planner's problem and the force commander's options. In addition to the threat from the opposing force, the field commander will face structural damage, local industrial hazards, and loss of mobility and degradation of communication links.

Combined, the future battlefield and force deployment scenarios will, in spite of extensive training, provide for extremely high levels of stress. The threats from emerging bacteria and viruses, chemical weapons and industrial compounds, and the urban battlefield will additionally inhibit and stress combat forces. Changes in force structure, national demographics, and the greater reliance on women in combat roles will require minimal changes in force protection.

Natural disease or disease from biological or chemical weapons, non-battle injury, including industrial-hazard exposure, and stress will continue to be the major threats to deployed forces in the future. Military and industrial intelligence of contested areas, modern equipment, extensive training, and pre- and post-deployment health studies will provide the most successful means of force protection.

The Nature of Risk Assessment and its Application to Deployed Forces

Joseph V. Rodricks, Ph.D.
The Life Sciences Consultancy, Washington, DC

Abstract

An analytical framework applicable to the assessment of the wide range of risks to health and safety potentially encountered by U.S. forces deployed to unfamiliar environments is presented as a guide to experts involved in the evaluation of diverse information on specific hazards. Adherence to the guidance should ensure that risk assessment results are clearly and consistently presented, and that they are suitable for practical, risk-management decision-making. The analytical framework presented is that first described by the National Research Council (NRC) (1983) and long in use for assessing risks of hazardous conditions, substances, and agents (referred to collectively as "stressors"). This paper attempts to describe how the analytical framework can be applied in diverse situations, and to many types of stressors, such as pathogens, toxic chemicals, and physical hazards. The framework for risk assessment, as originally conceived by the NRC, is a guide to the organization and evaluation of information and its attendant uncertainties, and does not require specific methodological approaches; the methodologies used should be those appropriate to the relevant scientific disciplines (e.g., toxicology, microbiology). The framework offered in the paper includes a means for reduction of complex information to usable formats. It recognizes that the purpose of the risk-assessment process is *not* to set standards that can be used for "yes-no" decision-making. Rather, in the current context, its purpose is to allow the Department of Defense decision-makers sufficient information to examine a range of risks that might arise in rapidly changing deployment conditions, and to balance competing risks so that overall risks to deployed forces can be minimized.

Future Health Assessment and Risk Management Integration for Infectious Diseases and Biological Weapons for Deployed U.S. Forces

Joan Rose, Ph.D.
University of South Florida, St. Petersburg, FL

Abstract

The health of the United States armed forces has been viewed as a critical component of the strength, readiness, and effectiveness of the military's ability to meet various degrees of threats to peace, human rights abuses, and other global disasters in the United States and the world. Compared with any other country or entity in the world, the U.S. military has one of the best surveillance and monitoring systems for assessing the risk of infectious disease globally. The monitoring is broad-based, specific for a large list of pathogenic agents, but includes generic symptomology that might be due to a multitude of current, emerging, or reemerging microorganisms; the monitoring is also timely. Gastrointestinal illness and respiratory and skin infections remain a problem for deployed troops.

It is now well known that microbial infections can result in chronic outcomes associated with heart, neurological, and immunological disorders. Therefore, hospitalization data will no longer suffice as the sole measure of severity and lost effectiveness to the troop force at large. Better assessment of antibiotic-resistant bacteria, coxsackieviruses, and *Legionella* and an evaluation of the underdiagnosis and underreporting of protozoa such as *Cryptosporidium* are needed. New microorganisms are being reported every year that might be associated with many of these illnesses, and prospective surveillance might be needed using new techniques to better understand the infection rates and asymptomatic infections.

Risk-assessment methods can now be used to quantify the risk of microbial infections and to address exposure and potential outcome from naturally occurring microorganisms and biological weapons. Hazard identification includes the identification of the microbial agent as well as the spectrum of human illnesses ranging from asymptomatic infections to death. The host response to the microorganisms with regard to immunity and multiple exposures should be addressed here, as well as the adequacy of animal models for studying human impacts. Endemic and epidemic disease investigations, case studies, hospitalization studies, and other epidemiological data are needed to complete this step in the risk assessment. The variables need to be carefully defined and the data quantified as ratios. The dose-response assessment is the mathematical characterization of the relationship between the dose administered and the probability of infection or disease in the exposed population. Dose-response assessments have been referred to as probability-of-infection models, which are developed from mostly human volunteer studies. The exposure assessment determines the size and nature of the population exposed, the route, concentrations, and distribution of the microorganisms, and the duration of the exposure. The description of exposure includes not only occurrence based on concentrations but also the prevalence (how often the microorganisms are found) and distribution of microorganisms in space and over time. Exposure assessment is determined through occurrence monitoring and predictive microbiology. Quantitative risk characterization should estimate the magnitude of the public health problem, and demonstrate the variability and uncertainty of the hazard, using four distributions: (1) the spectrum of health outcomes; (2) the confidence limits surrounding the dose-response model; (3) the distribution of the occurrence of the microorganism; and (4) the exposure distribution. Assessments of occurrence and exposure can be further delineated by distributions surrounding the method of recovery and survival (treatment) distributions.

The risk-assessment framework already fits into the Department of Defense's (DOD's) programs associated with risk management. The critical need will be the development of databases that can be used in the decision and management process. Although health outcomes and morbidity and mortality statistics are available from numerous databases and surveillance programs, the data lacking are often the long-term assessments and chronic outcomes. The exposure assessment, particularly during deployment, is more suspect to uncertainty, especially in terms of quantitative evaluations. Geographic, climatic, seasonal, dose-response, and exposure scenarios can be used to develop tools for setting priorities for assessment of pre-deployment risks. Risk models can be evaluated for plausibility during outbreak investigations or disease surveillance operations. Exposure and health outcomes must be better assessed.

The use of quantitative assessments allows one to begin to build exposure scenarios in which thresholds associated with ineffectiveness in the troops in a given time frame can be determined for specific agents. For biological weapons, dose-response models should be developed and time and concentration exposure and consequence scenarios should be built and evaluated.

Finally, the formal expansion of DOD's mission on emerging infectious diseases in June 1996 by Presidential Decision Directive NSTC-7 now includes global surveillance, training, research, and response. One of the major assets in implementing this new directive is the overseas research laboratory system that is currently in place: the DOD Infectious Disease Research Laboratories. At a minimum, each laboratory staff should be trained in risk-assessment methods, should have molecular capabilities (polymerase chain reaction [PCR]), and be trained in the use of the global information system (GIS) for maintaining and analyzing the databases.

Approaches for Using Toxicokinetic Information in Assessing Risk to Deployed U.S. Forces

Karl Rozman, Ph.D.
University of Kansas Medical Center, Kansas City, KS

Abstract

If there is no exposure, there is no toxicity. If there is exposure, toxicity might ensue when exposure exceeds a certain dose or time, a topic discussed under toxicokinetics and toxicodynamics. Analysis of the fundamental equation of toxicity yields the recognition of three independent time scales. One is the dynamic time scale, which is an intrinsic property of a given compound (what does a chemical do to an organism). The second is the kinetic time scale, which is an intrinsic property of a specific organism (what does an organism do to a chemical). The frequency of exposure denotes the third time scale, which is independent of dose and of the dynamic and kinetic time scales. Frequency of exposure depends on the experimental design or nature, but not on the organism or substance. A liminal condition occurs when the frequency becomes infinite, which corresponds to continuous exposure. Continuous exposure forces the dynamic and kinetic time scales to become synchronized, thereby reducing complexity to three variables: dose, effect, and one time scale. Keeping one of those variables constant allows one to study the other two variables reproducibly under isoeffective, isodosic, or isotemporal conditions. However, any departure from continuous exposure will introduce the full complexity of four independent variables (dose, and the kinetic, dynamic, and frequency time scales) impacting on the effect (dependent variable) at the same time. The examples discussed in this paper demonstrate how nature in the form of long half-lives provides liminal conditions when either kinetic or dynamic half-lives force synchronization of all three time scales.

The original charge for this paper was to conceptualize the role of toxicokinetics in the risk assessment of deployed forces exposed to chemicals. Most toxicologists familiar with current trends in toxicology are aware of the tremendous proliferation of publications combining physiologically based pharmacokinetic (PBPK) models with various dose-response extrapolation models, usually with the linearized multistage (LMS) model, or more recently with the benchmark (BM) curve-fitting approach. This author has used both PBPK and classical pharmacokinetics in many experiments. Although both are conceptually sound, there is one fundamental difference: classical pharmacokinetics uses time as an explicit function, whereas PBPK deals with time mostly as a variable, to be predicted based on physiological and physicochemical parameters. Therefore, the concepts of classical pharmacokinetics were helpful in the development of the initial core of a theory of toxicology, as presented in this document, whereas the concepts of PBPK were not as useful. This is not to say that combining PBPK with a theoretically sound biological model will not provide appropriate answers in some instances. However, as long as PBPK is used in conjunction with biologically implausible models (LMS, BM), it will lead (not surprisingly) to insignificant improvements. Central to the development of the concepts presented here was the notion that time is a variable equivalent to dose in toxicology. This idea has been around among toxicologists for almost exactly 100 years. Nevertheless, claims of exceptions to this idea as embodied in Haber's Rule prevented the development of time as a variable of toxicity. Even today toxicologists tend to focus on the so-called "exceptions" when effects are overwhelmingly dose—but not time—dependent. They do not realize that they are studying extreme parts of a spectrum under liminal conditions (e.g., a highly reversible effect on a short time scale), and they use experimental models with insufficient time resolution. When time resolution is satisfactory (such as pungency on a scale of seconds), clear summation effects emerge.

Recognition of the limits of the current risk-assessment paradigm made a paradox clear: none of the current risk projections include time as a variable even though any and all such risk predictions are by definition made in time. From this recognition it was concluded that something that is basically flawed cannot be fixed. Therefore, a new risk-assessment paradigm that includes time as a variable of toxicity, is being suggested. It is clear that although dose is a simple function (number of molecules), time is a complex variable, which runs on many different scales, at least three of which are interacting with dose to provide the complexity that seems to have bewildered generations of toxicologists. The three time scales are the toxicokinetic and toxicodynamic half-lives and the frequency of exposure. Thus, there are three liminal conditions:

1. When the toxicokinetic half-life is very long, it keeps the frequency of exposure essentially infinite (continuous exposure), and the toxicodynamic half-life by definition will be the same as the toxicokinetic one. Under these liminal conditions, $c \times t = k$ for isoeffective experiments, because there is only dose-dependence and one time-dependence.
2. When the toxicodynamic half-life is very long, it requires no additional injury to occur to keep injury constant nor the continuous presence of the noxious agent to result under isoeffective conditions in $c \times t = k$, because there is only dose- dependence and one time-dependence.
3. When the toxicokinetic/toxicodynamic half-lives become very short, they will blur the distinction between the kinetic and dynamic time scales and both will become less important, because in that case the frequency of exposure dominates the time-dependence. Under liminal (continuous exposure = infinite frequency) and isoeffective conditions, this will also lead to $c \times t = k$.

When experiments are conducted under isodosic or isotemporal conditions, then the relationship will obey the equation $c \times t = k \times \mathit{Effect}$. The vast majority of exposure scenarios are of course far from these liminal situations (ideal conditions) and will, therefore, yield $c \times t^x = k$. There are clear suggestions in this paper for the type of experiments that need to be done to determine x with exactitude. In the meantime, practical suggestions are included, which illustrate how to use a decision tree or available databases to conduct risk assessments for deployment situations that are less arbitrary by using both dose and time as variables of toxicity.

The decision tree approach uses a top-to-bottom analysis of identifying rate-determining or rate-limiting steps in the toxic action of a given compound for a specific effect. The advantage of this approach is its flexibility of determining at what level to contemplate modeling (risk assessment) of toxicity without having to rely on default assumptions. As recognized by other scientific disciplines, understanding of complexity is always advanced at three levels of investigations: experimental, computational, and theoretical. For the most part, toxicologists were and are engaged in experimental and computational studies with very little, if any, progress having been made in developing a comprehensive theory of toxicology. The combined theory and decision-tree analysis presented here should allow rapid progress in improving predictions of toxicity, if experimental design, computational goal, and theory come into equilibrium in terms of checks and balances. Instead of claiming exceptions, the three questions to be asked should be:

1. Why do some experimental results deviate from $c \times t = k$ (iso-effective) or $c \times t = k \times \mathit{Effect}$ (isodosic, isotemporal)?
2. What kind of computational (modeling) approach, and what level of integration, is needed to transform $c \times t^x = k$ or $c \times t^x = k \times \mathit{Effect}$ back to $c \times t = k$ or $c \times t = k \times \mathit{Effect}$?
3. How does exploration of Questions 1 and 2 improve the theory of toxicology, specifically the understanding of k?

It must be recognized that eventually experiments will be conducted under ideal conditions $c \times t = k$ or $c \times t = k \times \mathit{Effect}$). Once it is known how to transform $c \times t^x = k$ or $c \times t^x = k \times \mathit{Effect}$ (real-life situations) back to the ideal conditions, then any projection will also be possible in the opposite direction. Thus, it can be expected that the vast majority of experiments conducted under less-than-ideal conditions will then become interpretable by using a related study, which has been conducted under ideal conditions.

Health Risks and Preventive Research Strategy for Deployed U.S. Forces from Toxicologic Interactions Among Potentially Harmful Agents

Raymond Yang, Ph.D.
Colorado State University, Fort Collins, CO

Abstract

The goal of this paper is to recommend to the Department of Defense (DOD) a preventive research strategy for deployed U.S. forces to prevent future illness from toxicological interactions from potentially harmful agents. By doing so, it is implicit that potential health risks exist in deployments because of possible exposures to multiple chemicals, drugs, and biologics under stressful environmental and occupational conditions similar to those in the Persian Gulf War. This conclusion was reached based on the author's knowledge of toxicological interactions among chemicals and other agents and his assessment of the available literature information to date. It should be emphasized that this is not an effort to provide an exhaustive review of the field of toxicological interactions of chemical mixtures and other stressors. In fact, some of the areas are so new that the knowledge base is embryonic at best. DOD, through the National Research Council (NRC), seeks expert advice because of the limited information in the area of adverse health effects resulting from multiple stressors, including exposure to chemical mixtures, drug mixtures, vaccine mixtures, and physical and biological agents under highly stressful and hazardous environmental and occupational conditions. Furthermore, psychological stress undoubtedly plays a role in the potential development of such adverse health effects. There is probably no one individual or any group of individuals who knows the answers to such complex situations. Therefore, the author's opinions are, in some cases, based on educated guesses.

Given the principal goal stated above, this paper:

(1) Discusses the current thinking on toxicological interactions at low-exposure doses, principally to chemicals. However, known and potential toxicological interactions involving biological and physical agents, as well as stressful environmental conditions, are also discussed.

(2) Provides an assessment based on experimental toxicological studies of the effects of agents known to be present in the Persian Gulf War. The concerns about the surprising toxicological interactions discovered after the Persian Gulf War are discussed. These new discoveries offer potential explanations for the Gulf War Syndrome.

(3) Illustrates the importance of the mechanistic understanding of the disease process through research by summarizing some of the studies reported in the literature, which offers a possible explanation for the neurotoxicities of the Gulf War Syndrome.

(4) Looks into the rediscovered area of hormesis, as well as the little-known area of multiple stressors. Their potential roles in the field of toxicological interactions are discussed.

(5) Explains genetic polymorphism as a basis for sensitive populations. A specific example in experimental toxicology involving multiple stressors is given as an illustration.

(6) Offers a preventive research strategy to DOD to avoid possible future Gulf War Illnesses in deployed forces. The rationale, significance, and how-to's for such a preventive research strategy are given in detail.

(7) Discusses the ongoing and possible future development of predictive tools for toxicological interactions among chemicals, drugs, biologics, physical and biological agents, and other multiple stressors. Philosophical issues and future perspectives in the context of the present task are also discussed.

B

Biographical Information on Principal Investigator and Advisory Group

PRINCIPAL INVESTIGATOR

Lorenz Rhomberg is assistant professor of risk analysis and environmental health at the Harvard School of Public Health. He received his Ph.D. in biology from State University of New York at Stony Brook. His research interests focus on the development and critical analysis of more biologically based methods for human health risk assessment, especially on quantitative methods for cross-species extrapolation of toxic effects, comparative dosimetry, the use of biomarkers, and physiologically based pharmacokinetic modeling to address how measures of dose at the "target-organ" level relate to toxic effects across species and across variations in dosing regime. He has also developed methodologies for quantitative risk assessment of heritable genetic changes and examined the role of species-specific time scales in determining equivalent dose regimes in humans and experimental animals. Current projects focus on distributional representations of uncertainty factors in noncancer risk assessment.

ADVISORY GROUP

Arthur J. Barsky is a professor in the Department of Psychiatry at the Harvard Medical School and a psychiatrist at Brigham and Women's Hospital in Boston, where he supervises the Psychiatric Consultation Liaison Service and is the director of psychosomatic research. Dr. Barsky received an M.D. from Columbia University College of Physicians and Surgeons. His research interests include somatoform disorders, interindividual variability in symptom reporting among the medically ill, and psychiatric and psychosocial aspects of chronic medical illness.

Germaine M. Buck is an associate professor in the Department of Social and Preventive Medicine and an associate professor in the Departments of Gynecology-Obstetrics and Pediatrics, School of Medicine and Biomedical Sciences, State University of New York at Buffalo. She is also an adjunct associate professor in the Department of Epidemiology, School of Public Health, State University of New York at Albany. She received a Ph.D. in epidemiology from SUNY at Buffalo. Dr. Buck's research interests are in reproductive and perinatal outcomes, particularly following environmental exposures.

William S. Cain is a professor of surgery (otolaryngology) at the University of California School of Medicine in San Diego. He received a Ph.D. in experimental psychology from Brown University. His research areas include environmental health and physiology, chemosensory perception, and the acute health effect of exposure to chemicals.

John Doull is professor emeritus in the Department of Pharmacology, Toxicology and Therapeutics at the University of Kansas Medical Center. He received a Ph.D. in pharmacology and an M.D. from the University of Chicago. His research interests include general toxicology, toxicity of pesticides, and biological aspects of ionizing radiation.

Ernest Hodgson is the William Neal Reynolds Professor in the Department of Toxicology at North Carolina State University. He received a Ph.D. from Oregon State University. His research interests include enzymatic aspects of toxicology, comparative toxicology, and risk analysis. Dr. Hodgson has previously served on the NRC's Committee on Comparative Toxicity of Naturally Occurring Carcinogens.

David H. Moore is director of medical toxicology programs for Battelle Memorial Institute's Edgewood Operations. He received a Ph.D. in physiology from Emory University. He has been involved in elucidating the effects of nerve agents on airway smooth muscle, developing the concept of a topical skin protectant, and studying the pharmacokinetics of oximes and anticonvulsants for possible use in treating nerve agent poisoning.

Roy Reuter is vice president of Life Systems, Inc. He oversees environmental and health effects research for governmental and private-sector clients. He has a Ph.D. in sanitary engineering and has over 40 years of experience working in the field of environmental engineering. Dr. Reuter has been involved in 18 major programs on cleanup, conservation, compliance, and pollution prevention for Army environmental offices and laboratories. He was involved in developing the Joint Deployment Toxicology Research and Development Program Plan. He has also been extensively involved in assessments of toxicological data, the collection and analysis of environmental information, and exposure hazard and risk assessments.

Ken W. Sexton is the Bond Professor of Environmental Health in the School of Public Health at the University of Minnesota. In addition, he is the director of the Center for Environment and Health Policy. He received a Sc.D. in environmental health sciences from Harvard University. His research interests include the role of science in environmental decision-making; assessment, management, and communication of environmental risks; evaluation of human exposures to toxic agents; and analysis of public policy related to environmental health.

Robert E. Shope is professor of pathology, microbiology and immunology, and preventive medicine and community health at the University of Texas at Galveston. He received an M.D. from Cornell University. His research interests include emerging infectious diseases and the epidemiology of arbovirus and rabies virus infections.

Ainsley Weston is team leader for molecular carcinogenesis at the National Institute for Occupational Safety and Health (NIOSH). He received a Ph.D. in carcinogen biochemistry from the University of London. His research interests include molecular epidemiology and the development of methods for the detection of genotoxicity and other dosimeters and markers of human internal exposure to carcinogens.